INTIMATE
MATTERS

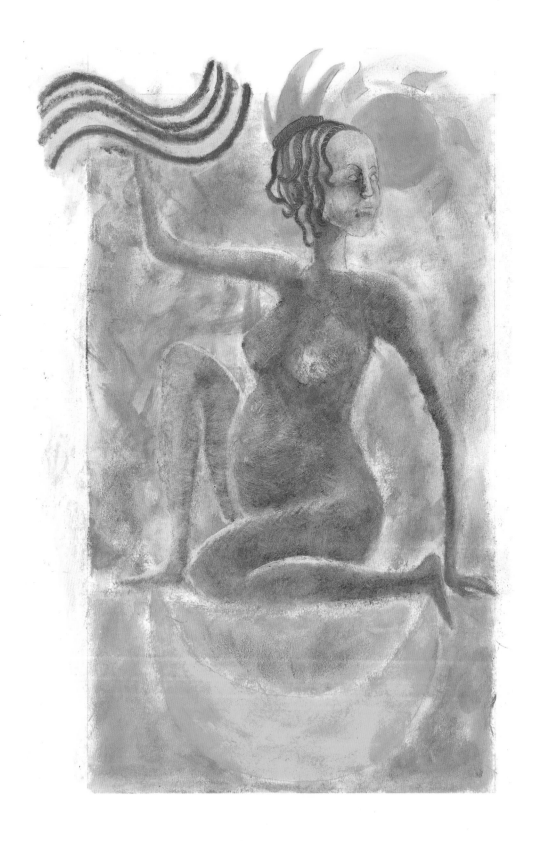

INTIMATE
MATTERS

Restoring balance and harmony
to the feminine experience

A GAIA ORIGINAL

Linda Valins

Gaia Books Limited

A GAIA ORIGINAL

Conceived by Linda Valins and Joss Pearson

Editorial: Fiona Trent

Design: Sara Mathews

Direction: Joss Pearson
Patrick Nugent
Joanna Godfrey Wood

Dedicated with love
to my mother, Julia,
and her precious
memories of my
dear father,
Nathan Bensusan
(1920 – 1991).

This is a Registered Trade Mark of Gaia Books Limited

First published in the United Kingdom in 1993
by Gaia Books Limited
66 Charlotte Street,   and   20 High Street, Stroud,
London, WIP 1LR   Glos GL5 1AS

Printed and bound by Mandarin Offset in Hong Kong
Colour reproduction by MRM Graphics Ltd, Winslow, Bucks, England
A catalogue record for this book is available from the British Library
ISBN 1 85675 070 1
10 9 8 7 6 5 4 3 2 1

Cover Illustration Giovanna Pierce

Foreword

Linda Valins' illuminating and delightful book *Intimate Matters* is, in many ways, about taking responsibility: for your own health, and for your relationships, not only with your partner, unborn baby, children, and health practitioners and yourself, but also with the environment, and in doing so improving the world for all of us.

Linda teaches and encourages you to get in touch and in tune with your body. Through inspiring exercises she helps you, for example, to concentrate on your breathing, using your breath and your own inner resources to bring a sense of harmony and wellbeing back into your life.

In any relationship there needs to be a balance, if one side of the partnership becomes too dominant both members will suffer. *Intimate Matters* attempts to redress the balance and to bring harmony back into women's health care. As a midwife I am well acquainted with the destructive influences that occur when the balance between male and female becomes too strong in one or other direction.

A common example of imbalance is when obstetricians rule the roost – midwives and women are cowed and the technology of childbirth sometimes seems to be used as an assault against the expectant mother, "saving the baby" from its mother's "dangerous" and "destructive" body. When the feminine and masculine are in balance in a maternity unit, and there is mutual respect between midwives, obstetricians, and the birthing women, the women who give birth feel empowered by the whole experience.

One of Linda's strongest messages is that of communication. As a midwife who talks to babies inside the uterus to let them know that they are safe, to ensure them of a welcome to the world, I love the suggestions and examples Linda gives of gentle communication between surgeon and unconscious patient, between the healer and the woman who is healed.

Thank you Linda for your lovely book.

Caroline Flint SRN SCM ADM

CONTENTS

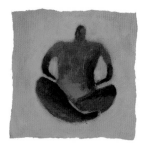
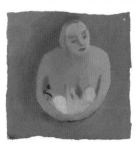
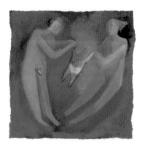

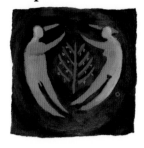
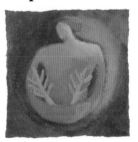
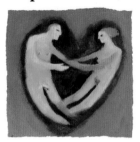
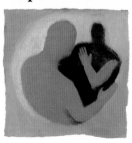

Introduction

I was nervous and alarmed. For several weeks I had been experiencing unexplained bleeding outside my menstrual period, and wondered what was causing it. Was it an early menopause (I was 37) – or something more serious? I knew little about the workings of my body, and even less about appropriate treatments. By good fortune I was recommended to a gynaecologist whose advice was to wait, and not to intervene by prescribing drugs or undertaking investigative surgery. His approach was not, however, based on complacency or ignorance, but rather on experience gained through his intuitive and trusting awareness of the natural rhythms of the female body. The gynaecologist was able to adopt this non-interventionist, sensitive approach after learning that two weeks previously my much-loved grandmother had died. He sensed that my body was reacting to the grief I was feeling, and he felt no need to take direct action at this stage. This approach may be described as working from the feminine perspective in health care.

WHAT THIS BOOK IS ABOUT

At some point in every woman's life she will visit a gynaecologist. Unlike men, women visit doctors not only during ill health but also, for example, to arrange contraception, or for care during pregnancy. Such visits often involve the women being examined intimately, and by their very nature, encroach on various aspects of a woman's self: biological, sexual, emotional, and spiritual.

Although this is a universal female experience, the issues surrounding gynaecology are rarely written about from the feminine perspective – from the receiver's rather than from the health practitioner's perspective.

Through the combined efforts of the women's movement and feminism, much has been discussed, written about, and to some extent, achieved, to improve the role of women in society. Yet, when a woman enters her doctor's surgery, it can often feel as if she has been transported back to the nineteenth century. She becomes passive and feels vulnerable. She is enveloped in the male-dominated culture of medicine, which tends to view her in "bits", rather than as a whole person, and dismisses her experience of being a woman.

Alternative therapies are currently enjoying renewed interest, partly because of an increasing dissatisfaction with orthodox (conventional) medicine. Holistic, or "whole person", therapies are concerned with restoring natural balance and harmony to the body by promoting our innate healing powers. This book is about creating a more positive experience between women and their bodies in order to help increase knowledge of our natural cycles and thereby improve health. It aims to demystify what happens inside a woman's body, and concentrates on prevention through awareness rather than cure.

AN IMBALANCE OF FEMININE AND MASCULINE CAUSES PROBLEMS IN HEALTH AND NATURE

The very essence of being "whole" and healthy depends on our recognition of the male and female aspects that exist in every one of us. Feminine qualities are not just confined to women, nor are masculine qualities just confined to men. They are aspects in all of us that need to be understood, developed, and most importantly, balanced.

Feminine qualities embody intuition, nurturing, and compassion, and represent the "feeling" and creative sides of our nature. The feminine principle is to honour the Earth, to feel a part of her. The masculine principle is symbolized in our culture by rulership and power, will, vitality, and intellect.

A dominance of the masculine over the feminine – or the feminine over the masculine – may create disharmony and dis-ease. The manifestation of feminine and spiritual values in medicine is critical, not only for our health, but for our homes, and our planet. By restoring the feminine principle into our lives we will have begun the process of re-integrating mind, body, and spirit into medicine.

THE "SUPERMAN" PRINCIPLE

These ideas and concerns sprang from numerous letters I received from women who wrote to me after reading my first book on vaginismus – a condition whereby the vagina contracts involuntarily to prevent intercourse. Although I was prepared to hear from vaginismus sufferers, I was totally unprepared to hear from non-sufferers, who as a last resort, wrote to me hoping I would be able to help them with their gynaecological problems. Many described unsatisfactory treatments and experiences with doctors, and those who had sought help from alternative practitioners had not faired much better.

Slowly I began to see the emergence of a common theme. It seemed that the masculine principle had become so dominant in the healing relationship that it had led the practitioners – conventional and alternative – not only to deny and invalidate their patient's intuition and inner knowledge about her own body, but also their own.

This has partly happened as a result of the over dominance in our culture of the "Superman principle", which sees illness as something that must be conquered and eradicated, without viewing symptoms as bodily expressions of emotional or spiritual conflicts.

Five weeks before I began to write this book I experienced a major loss in my life. My father died unexpectedly, which filled me with grief, and a void that expresses itself in our family as a tangible imbalance. He died as the result of a highly toxic drug, which had been prescribed to alleviate rheumatoid arthritis. A drug that is usually given to cancer patients to destroy their tumours destroyed my father's healthy cells, and he finally suffered a heart attack.

It struck me that although he was a man, the masculine side of his nature, which might have questioned and objected to such a treatment, did not emerge. Had my father been encouraged to become more aware, assertive, intuitive, and trusting of his own body, he may have been less willing to have been the passive recipient of such a dangerous drug.

The masculine-oriented state of Western health care is not, however, just men's doing. Women physicians and scientists, acting from the masculine principle often become more male and interventionist. Jeanne Achterberg believes the answer is not in getting female doctors to dominate

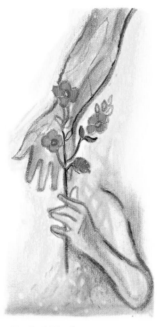

Herbal Healer
The relationship between midwife and birthing woman was the first healing partnership: based on trust, respect, and equality.

The cycle of life
"Our cycle is like the cycle of a plant. There is a right time for planting the seed , for growing and branching out, for letting go of the seed and for coming back into our own roots of ourselves."
ANNIE SHAW

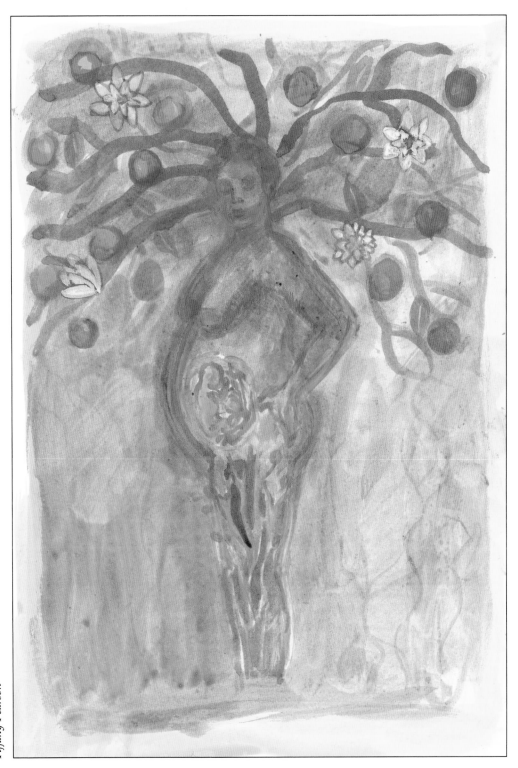

Tiffany Pearson

medicine, but rather to enable both men and women, as receivers and givers of health care, to become more aware of their masculine and feminine qualities in order to help develop, integrate, and balance them. The major theme of this book is the belief that restoring feminine principles to health care can be a positive and healing experience, not just for the patient but also for the health practitioner.

ON YOUR OWN OR TOGETHER?

Throughout this book, when I am addressing issues that relate to you and your lover, I refer to partners. This is not meant to exclude anyone who does not have a partner. It is quite acceptable not to be with someone. Feeling that it is somehow "wrong" to be without a partner can be very destructive. It creates desperation and forces people to enter bad relationships and stay in unhealthy ones.

Even if you are not currently with a partner, give space to yourself for the possibility of having loving relationships. Ultimately, the most important relationship of your life is with yourself, and when that heals then the opportunity and possibility of forming a relationship with someone else increases.

HOW THIS BOOK WILL ENHANCE YOUR HEALTH

One of the most difficult and unexplored relationships many women encounter is with their own body image. Many of us feel either too fat, too thin, too tall, too short, or generally not beautiful enough. Unconsciously women tend to be cruel to their bodies, as demonstrated in the use of cosmetic surgery and drastic diet regimes. We often feel insecure, unhappy, and frightened about our bodies. This book can help a woman to relate to her body as a temple, honouring and uniting the spiritual and physical.

Through practical and spiritual exercises, this book will take you beyond conceptual thinking, to achieve body-mind harmony. The ideas presented here will enable you to:

- Explore the menstrual cycle as a source of creativity, spirituality, and inner knowledge
- Prevent infertility through awareness

- Promote fertility through consciousness
- Deepen your lovemaking
- Enhance your sexuality
- Understand and improve your health through your relationship with your health practitioner
- Become aware of and bring into balance and flow your feminine and masculine sides
- Become more conscious and maintain good health

This book is highly practical and non-medical. It explores feelings, not just facts; experiences, not just theories. The aim of this book is to explore and understand the spiritual and emotional aspects of health, therefore purely clinical details are rarely focused upon. While knowledge of one's anatomy is helpful, it does not have to be acquired from dissecting bodies or studying medical texts. You can become intimately knowlegeable about your body through experiencing it from within by developing awareness of your emotions, thoughts, body, and speech.

Restoring feminine and spiritual values into health care means combining art with science, caring with curing, knowledge with intuition, and intervention with love. This can be achieved by inspiring women, their partners, and health professionals to reclaim the inner wisdom that many of us feel has been lost, in order to help improve the quality of our health, our lives and the planet.

Health is related to something deeply spiritual, and I hope that you will discover this from my book.

Linda Valins
London
Summer 1992

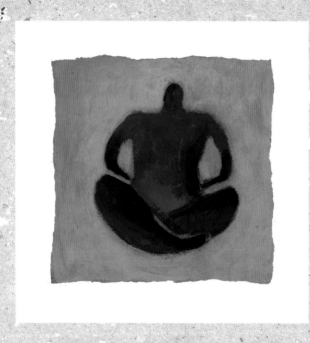

CHAPTER 1

THE FEMININE AND
THE MASCULINE

*"Few words are so revealing of Western sexual prejudice as the word
Goddess, in contrast to the word God. Modern connotations vastly differ
from those of the ancients, to whom the Goddess was a full-fledged cosmic
parent figure who created the universe and its laws. . ."*
BARBARA WALKER, THE WOMAN'S ENCYCLOPEDIA OF
MYTHS AND SECRETS

In 1527 Paracelsus, considered one of the greatest physicians of his time, burned his official pharmacopoeia declaring that "he had learned from the Sorceresses all that he knew". Who were these women, and how did they come to gain such valuable insights into holistic healing?

Women have always possessed an innate knowledge of their bodies and the power to heal. Indeed, for much of human pre-history, women and the life-force were revered. The image of woman as goddess originated from her menstrual cycle, where women's ability to bleed each month, and their potential for pregnancy and birth, was seen as their oneness with Mother Earth and the goddess' lunar cycle. Even after women-centred society – matriarchy – gave way to male-centred civilizations, women's special healing ability and connection with birth, life, and death persisted in folk culture.

This early reverence of woman as "goddess of creation" has now vanished, and as a result, many women have lost their connection with Nature, an awareness of and respect for their natural bodily functions and cycles, and thereby also the power to heal themselves.

The demise of the feminine in women's health care

In the Western, post-classical world, the application of women's wisdom and intuitive methods of healing came to a violent and abrupt end in the Middle Ages. Men, through envy and fear, a sense of exclusion and powerlessness, mis-interpreted women's healing skill through knowledge of their cycles, their bodies, herbs, and the moon's phases, as signs of supernatural and dark powers. As a consequence, towns and villages throughout Europe witnessed witch hunts: the ritual burning of some nine million women. Perhaps the over-reverence of women as "goddesses", without the inclusion of men as gods, had led to the destructive notion that one sex was superior to the other.

As the feminine principle was slowly destroyed, the way was opened up for male-oriented religions, societies, and the beginnings of orthodox (conventional) medicine. Combined with the mass destruction of much of women's feminine knowledge came the dominance of Judeo-Christian images of a male, masterful God. The goddess was no longer part of accepted religion.

In women's health care the legacy of the demise of the feminine is still with us, as seen in mainstream medicine's opposition to – and repression of – holistic healing.

It sometimes seems that the medical profession seeks to control people's minds and bodies. This tendency is possi-bly unconscious, and probably originates from the powerlessness that people feel over their own lives and destinies. Nevertheless, this has had a devastating effect on the way in which women's disorders are treated within the specialties of psychiatry and gynaecology.

Cultural ideas about "proper" feminine behaviour have shaped the definition and treatment of female insanity for 150 years. Female insanity was specifically linked to what were perceived as the biological "crises" of the female life cycle: puberty, pregnancy, childbirth, and menopause. Doctors believed that during these so-called "crises" a

Assault against women
Women continue to be the major recipients and suffer-ers of masculine-oriented medicine, as demonstrated by the following British and American studies:
• *Thousands of mastectomies – surgical removal of one or both breasts – were performed on breast cancer patients before it was realized that it prob-ably offers no proven greater survival rate*
• *Over half of caesareans and hysterectomies are found to be unnecessary, particularly in the USA*
• *Many gynaecological procedures are dehumaniz-ing; most have not decreased mortality rates*
• *Women are twice as likely to be prescribed drugs than men with similar psycho-logical symptoms*
• *Women see doctors more often, and are admitted into hospitals – particularly psychiatric ones – in greater proportions than men*

woman's mind would be weakened, and the symptoms of insanity might emerge. In the nineteenth century this connection between women's seasons and their emotional states led to a distinct set of mental illnesses that had no male equivalents. The disorder known as "hysteria" was for centuries the quintessential female malady. The word is derived from the Greek "hysteron" (womb), and between 1870 and World War I it assumed a central role in female psychiatry. By the beginning of 1900 the word "hysterical" had become almost synonymous with "feminine", meaning all extremes of emotionality. Hysteria was linked to a vast repertoire of emotional and physical symptoms – fits, fainting, sobbing, paralysis, refusal to eat – and its unpredictability was associated with the feminine nature.

In the 1800s women who were diagnosed as mentally ill underwent immense suffering through the horrors of psychiatry and gynaecology. Many treatments for women's emotional disorders included gynaecological surgery, as in the removal of clitorides and ovaries, and brain operations such as "lobotomy" – surgical incision into the brain. In the 1940s, one North American neurologist lobotomized thirty-five women in one afternoon. Even today, women undergo more psychiatric interventions than men: in the United Kingdom and North America, women as Electro Convulsive Therapy (ECT) patients outnumber men by a ratio of two or even three to one (see also box on p. 16).

Since the 1970s and the advent of the Women's Liberation Movement, people have begun to challenge traditional psychoanalysis, psychiatry, obstetrics, and gynaecology, creating alternatives such as feminist therapy, natural birthing, and women's self-help health groups. However, in some ways this may have unwittingly polarized the issues further into a "feminist war", since all medical treatment – for both women and men of all ages, creeds, and colours – needs to be humanized.

THE GODDESS IN EVERY WOMAN

What was once called "witchcraft" is actually "womancraft": owning and understanding our own bodies, and being in charge of our own health. A central concern of feminist consciousness-raising groups has been to ensure that women know more about themselves from the point of view of feminine experience, and not from that of the prevailing masculine stereotype.

All the traditional goddess-names have their root meanings in the words "womb" or "vulva". The goddess simply means the feminine principle within every woman. To "make a friend of the goddess" is to "make a friend of one's womb". If you become aware of your bodily rhythms and feminine functions you are already beginning to harmonize with Nature: uniting the inner self and the outer world.

The moon and its goddesses have, at all times and in all cultures, been regarded as the quintessential image through which a woman may strengthen her sense of her own nature. If you recognize that the all-powerful fate to enhance your health and wellbeing is not wielded by some outside power, but exists in you and has enormous potential, then you will feel very differently about your body.

Knowledge of your body's rhythms and how to enhance your wellbeing is available to you now.

HOW TO RECLAIM YOUR INNER FEMININE KNOWLEDGE
- Look inward with trust
- Identify with goddesses' names, and what they represent
- Do not be afraid to learn from yourself and other women, rather than from medical books or doctors
- Recognize the "Gaia concept", the idea that the Earth is a unified living thing, and that what is done to any part, animal, or human being, affects us all
- Acknowledge that women and men are in this healing process together. Men suffer too. We are all interconnected – part of a whole – and therefore both sexes must join together and celebrate one another. There are differences between us, but our concern should be to celebrate the spirituality in both sexes, which transcends gender.

Partnership and strength
The feminine and the masculine can never exist in total isolation from each other. The Fonteyn-Nureyev partnership was one of harmonious unity. When they danced, they blended together as different aspects of the same whole, rather than as two opposing forces.

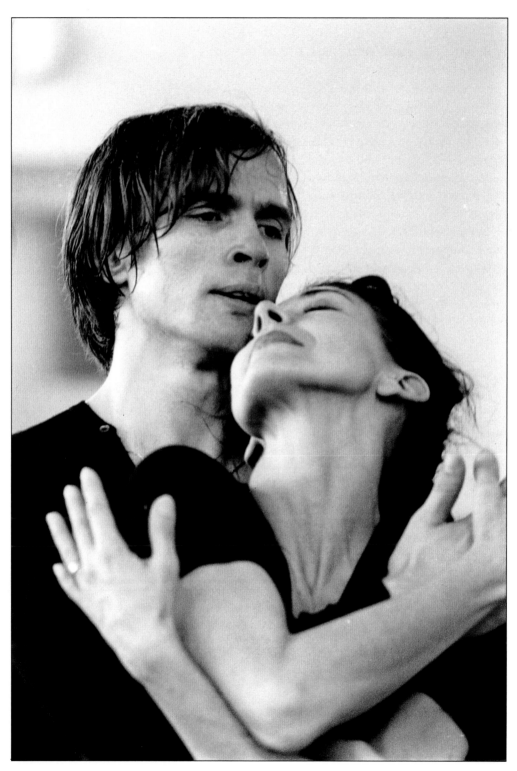

Frederika Vivian

A new appraisal of feminine and masculine

The Women's Movement of the late 1960s and '70s legiti-mately began to redress many sexual injustices and inequalities. If, however, any one aspect – female or male – becomes polarized or dominant, for example, female syn-onymous with "good" and male synonymous with "bad", this leads to dis-harmony and dis-ease. It is important not to get stuck in the terms "masculine" and "feminine"; we are really talking about balance and flow.

The abuse of men should also be recognized. In strict religious cultures, where male sexuality and the expression of emotion is repressed, the only release for men is often in the sexual/aggressive sphere. Patriarchy – male-centred society – may have been a backlash against matriarchy, indicating that women-centred societies may have been as unequal as our current male-centred culture.

ANIMUS AND ANIMA

Subtle stereotyping of sex roles teaches boys to be boys and girls not to be. Such conditioning has the effect that girls and boys come to accept certain characteristics as their own, and eliminate others that they do not feel to be theirs.

As a boy the Swiss psychoanalyst C. G. Jung noticed, and was fascinated by, the changing aspects of his mother, particularly during menstruation. He came to base his the-ory of "inner woman, inner man" on this discovery, and named them animus (Latin, "spirit") for the unconscious, masculine side of a woman's personality, and anima (Latin, "soul") for the unconscious, feminine side of a man's per-sonality. Jung believed that a connection with – and balance of – the feminine and masculine is essential for one's mental and physical wellbeing. The feminine is the receptive principle; the masculine goes out in the world and is active. Nothing is static, we need both principles to allow the flow of the natural life-force.

Jung did not mean that we are half male or half female, but rather that a woman's animus – the masculine side of her – allows her to push through to the outside world.

"[Women's and men's] obliga-tion is to describe masculine in such a way that it does not exclude the masculine in women, and yet hits a resonant string in the man's heart. Our obligation is to describe the feminine in a way that does not exclude the feminine in men but makes a large string resonate in the woman's heart."
ROBERT BLY, *IRON JOHN*

"The mistake we often make is to confuse the terms 'feminine' with women, and 'masculine' with men. Feminine qualities do not have to be epitomized by a woman, nor masculine by a man."
LYNN OSBORNE, ACUPUNC-TURIST AND OCCUPATIONAL THERAPIST

The feminine side of a man represents his receptivity, nurturing, and intuitive capacities. A man could use his anima – his tender side – to become interested in dance, or gardening. Or he could be the strong, outdoors type, like the character, "Crocodile Dundee", who is tough and "streetwise", but who also has a very sensitive nature.

Children learn aspects of the animus and anima from their parents. For example, a boy can tune in to his intuitive, gentle side from experiences such as going fishing with his father. Or a boy's inner woman may embody the ways in which he experiences his mother, which can affect his future relationships with other women. If a girl's animus is based on her father's unreliability and inconsistency, she may not develop a positive relationship with her own inner man. This may cause her to distance herself from either her masculine out-going qualities, or even from men themselves.

ANIMUS AND ANIMA IN INTIMATE HEALTH

Every woman holds, within her psyche, the masculine principle, though it may be very repressed. Fundamental to a woman's health is that she recognizes when her feminine side is dominant and her masculine side underdeveloped. If you are operating solely from your feminine side you may be over-vulnerable to being emotionally hurt. Connecting up with your animus can help you to protect and defend yourself. By strengthening the masculine side of yourself, you can become less open to exploitation, to unsuitable partnerships, and to consequent heartache. Some of the more obvious ways you can strengthen your animus are for example by becoming financially independent, and asserting yourself through a career.

If a woman over-identifies with her animus, she may drive her body flat out, like a machine at full throttle, until she burns out. If you do not make contact with your feminine side, particularly during menstruation, you will not allow yourself the necessary periods of rest and passivity, introspection, and relaxation.

21

THE MASCULINE AND FEMININE IN STORIES AND MYTHS

Many fairy tales illustrate the darkness and light in women, personified by the Fairy Godmother and the Bad Witch, and are wonderful ways in which to illustrate the psychological conflicts and unconscious fantasies related to childhood development.

Some tales illustrate animus possession in terms of a woman imprisoned in a tower. The story of Rapunzel symbolizes the point at which a woman is out of touch with the earth or feminine principle. Rapunzel is too "high" and ungrounded – in her tower – through overintellectualization. She can be seen as being overtaken by her inner male, not because she is intelligent, but because her energy is not balanced by a connection with Nature. Rapunzel's solution comes through a symbol of her connection to Nature, and her ability to relate in an embodied way. Her long blonde hair allows her to be rescued. In other stories, such as Sleeping Beauty and Snow White, help often comes in the form of a healthy, earthy male.

Perhaps you are a modern Rapunzel: you work hard and are too intellectually bound-up; you never relax. At night you bring work home, or clean your already spotless home. You ignore your connection to Nature and your body signals of fatigue and the need for rest. Eventually you may have to take notice and respond to Nature's call to free yourself from your intellect (your animus).

The following exercises can help raise your awareness of differences and similarities between men and women. If we are aware of stereotypes and prejudices – the dark side – we can come through to the light. The exercises illustrate how we can be mirrors for each other and recognize our polarized views of our sexuality.

EXERCISES TO EXPLORE SEXUAL STEREOTYPES.

The first explores stereotyped roles for women and men, and how these contrast with our feelings. The second helps us learn what sexual stereotypes mean to us, so that we are able to escape from them.

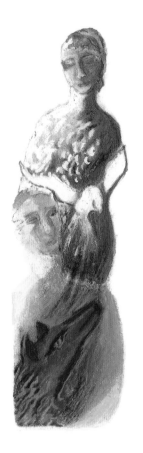

Animus and anima
Allowing and expressing the feminine within the man and the masculine within the woman ensures that the two animus and anima principles become less polarized. We need both principles alive and balanced within us to allow the flow of the natural life force.

• With a male partner (or friend) sit on the floor facing each other, and hold hands if you wish
• Keep eye contact
• In your turn start by saying sentences that begin, "As a woman I am expected to. . ." For example, "As a woman I am expected to be quiet", "As a woman I am expected to be passive", and so on
• After a few minutes change to sentences that begin, "As a woman I feel. . . angry, lonely. . ."
• Then swap roles
• Your partner might begin by saying, "As a man I am expected to succeed", or, "As a man I feel pressurized to be brave"
At the end share some feedback with your partner. Did he have similar experiences? What were the hardest expectations?
• With a partner, decide which of you will play the man, and which the woman
• Spend five minutes acting out these roles using movement, gesture, and words
• Change roles
• After ten minutes stop and spend five more minutes talking about what happened for both of you. Ask yourselves whether you noticed any differences in the way you moved, looked, the words you used, and how you saw the other person

MEDICINE: EAST AND WEST

Orthodox (allopathic) medicine dominates medical practice in the West. Allopathy means "to treat sickness oppositely", that is, to give medication that may counteract a symptom by causing an opposite reaction: treating diarrhoea with a drug that slows the intestines for example, or treating asthma with medicine that dilates the bronchial tubes. Homeopathy does the reverse. It treats "like with like", utilizing the principle that whatever can harm can also cure. A homeopath treats a condition with minute doses of a substance that would, in larger quantities, produce the same symptoms in a healthy person, seeking thereby to stimulate the body's own healing response.

Conventional medicine also tends to view disease as the mechanical breakdown of parts, organs, or systems. This is in direct contrast to the holistic method, which is based on the idea that no single part or symptom can be understood or healed except in its relation to the whole person.

To rediscover the principles of a more balanced way of caring for our bodies, such as existed before the witch hunts in Europe and North America, we have to look to China, where holistic medicine, reflecting our links with Nature, has survived and prospered.

The Chinese believe that it is basically more natural to be healthy than sick, which is why they used to pay their doctor only when he kept them healthy – the opposite to Western pracitice. Doctors in the West are trained in sickness, not health. The traditional healers of Ancient Greece, China, and India, unlike Western doctors, did not consider individuals' organs or emotions to be independent of their owner, or of the other people around them, or of the planet.

The human being in balance and flow

Balance and harmony are integral to traditional Chinese medicine. Their importance originates from the belief that Nature is seen as a whole, of which both women and men are an integral part. The word to describe this approach to life comes from the ancient Chinese cosmic religion known as "the Tao". The Tao is a difficult word to translate exactly since it is considered indefinable, but the closest translation is "the Way". The relevance of the Tao in health care is simply to describe the concepts of balanced living.

Enjoying good physical, spiritual, and emotional health relies on recognizing the power of maintaining a balance in everything that we do. Dis-ease is often the result of disharmony and imbalance in our mind-body. If we eat too many fatty foods, for example, we may gain unwanted weight because our body is being subjected to an imbalanced diet. Similarly, if we experience too much of the male or female

Umbrella titles for the different approaches to health care
- *Alternative Implies other than, or different from, what is conventionally on offer in (allopathic) orthodox practice.*
- *Natural Healing Refers to therapies devised before the advent of modern medicine, belonging to traditional societies, and taken direct from Nature.*
- *Holistic A philosophy rather than a therapy, which has a person-centred rather than a disease-focused approach. A holistic practitioner looks at the person as a whole, rather than as a series of parts.*
- *Complementary This is the most appropriate and well-known term, since it implies bridging the gap between mainstream and alternative approaches. Most therapies can complement whatever treatment your doctor may prescribe: integration is the key.*

The yin-yang theory
This is illustrated in the tradi-
tional black and white Chinese
Taoist symbol, which
represents harmonious unity.
It shows the two great forces
of the universe, the dark and
light, negative and positive,
female and male, to be held in
complete balance and equality
of power. There is a spot of
black in the white, and white in
the black, which is essential to
the symbolism, since there is
no being that does not contain
within itself the germ of its
opposite.

Yin and yang represent a
harmonious unity, because
everything has both a yin and
yang aspect. They are not two
opposing forces, but are differ-
ent aspects of the whole, two
sides of the same coin. The
feminine and masculine can
never exist in total isolation
from one another.

elements in our lives, our bodies may respond to the imbalance with emotional or physical symptoms.

YIN-YANG

Over two thousand years ago in China, the Yellow Emperor Huang Ti described a balance between two contrasting forces. One – known as yin – was described as dark, moist, watery, and female, while the other – called yang – was hot, dry, fiery, and male. In traditional Chinese medicine, the organs of the body are divided according to these feminine and masculine principles, and are seen as either predominantly yin or yang. Health is understood to be a happy harmony between these two forces, and disease is seen as evidence of disharmony, or a lack of balance.

Changes in the balance of these two opposing forces are normal. On some days you may feel fiery and assertive, and on others, a bit low and "under the weather". It is only when the balance becomes seriously disturbed that you actually become ill. The feminine (yin) and masculine (yang) principles can best be understood within the concepts of a holistic method of healing, such as acupuncture.

CASE STUDY: TANYA AND THE ACUPUNCTURIST

Tanya was suffering from stress after separating from her husband. Through sleeplessness and tension, her energies had become alarmingly depleted and her body reacted by expressing this in bouts of migraine, pre-menstrual tenderness in her breasts, and irregular monthly cycles. She sought the advice of an acupuncturist who specialized in women's health. It was through her that Tanya experienced the powerful healing of this ancient medical practice.

The acupuncturist's method of treating Tanya addressed not only the symptoms but her overall wellbeing. Her complete personal history was taken in minute detail, including many aspects of her menstrual cycle, and was woven together until it formed a "pattern of disharmony".

Acupuncture consists of righting the balance between yin and yang by stimulating points on the body with fine needles. These points – meridians or channels – lie along invisible lines and conduct vital energy (Ch'i) through the body. Each organ has its own meridian and corresponds to a specific emotion. An excess or prolonged experience of a particular emotion can disturb the flow of energy from/to the corresponding organ to cause disease.

The acupuncturist examined Tanya to see where the imbalances lay and diagnosed liver Ch'i stagnation. The liver is the most temperamental organ – easily affected by stress – and its function is to promote the smooth flow of Ch'i in all directions. By treating the appropriate points, the acupuncturist stimulated Tanya's meridians, which increased Tanya's energy flow and the innate healing properties in her body. The acupuncturist encouraged Tanya to direct her own attention to herself as a whole person, physically, emotionally, and spiritually.

Being in control

The possibility of increasing our psychic abilities is becoming an attractive idea to many people. Regrettably, the dark side of some current groups' philosophies use "psychic power" to intimidate, implying that we "should" be able to psychically "control" and "create" our own world – that we are wholly responsible, even to blame, for our destiny. The people who believe this forget that everyone is interconnected, and that no one is solely responsible for their own problems.

A different concept of control is a belief that the body has an integrity of its own, that it seeks health as its optimal state, and that in the normal course of events it maintains a fluctuating condition that can best be described as balance. Taking control of your health requires an acceptance of the fact that control in the conventional sense is not possible, and when you let go of control and trust your body you are beginning to harmonize with yourself and with Nature.

There is a tremendous difference between "psychic power" and increased awareness. In terms of health, relationships, and conception, increased awareness is about love, trust, self-development, responsibility, and co-operation – not competition – with Nature.

The Yin-yang family
The balance of a loving mother and father as caregivers (both female and male) is essential for a harmonious family environment, and for the wellbeing of a child's early development.

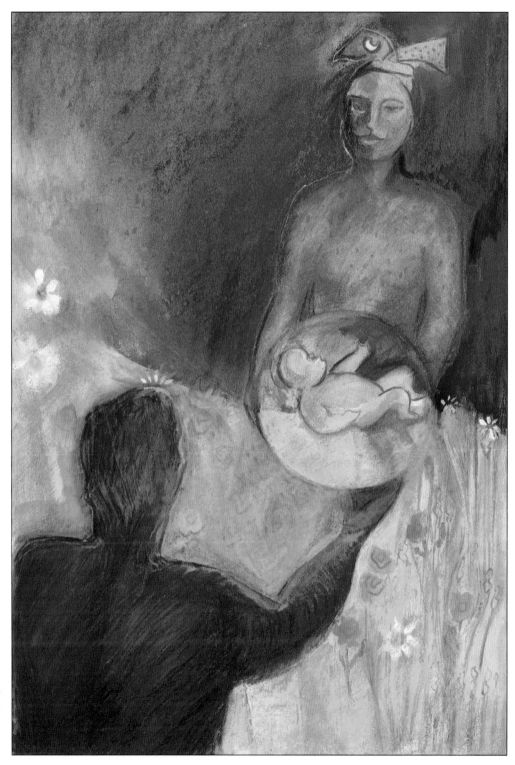

Sara Keeping

Of ourselves we can do nothing. You have no control over the mysteries of conception, birth, life, death, and the Universe: you have to lose control in order to find balance. What you can do however, is to become conscious and more responsible, through awareness of your breath, body, your thoughts and emotions, and your speech.

THE PRACTICE OF MINDFULNESS

It is often only when you become ill, or meet a life crisis, that you begin to reflect inwardly, and even then it may be difficult for you to see a connection between what is happening in your body and mind, and external events.

To maintain balance and flow between the feminine and masculine forces in your life, you must first become more "mindful". Mindfulness is usually associated with Zen Buddhist meditations. However, it is essentially practical and can provide the vital key in helping you stay emotionally, spiritually, and physically healthy. Mindfulness is to be awake and fully aware, to observe, and be attentive to, your breathing, body posture, emotions, thoughts, and speech. "To be present" means to relax with how, and who, you are. Meditation masters say: "When washing the dishes, wash the dishes", which simply means you need to stay with your present task, devote full attention to it, be fully aware of it from moment to moment, and not rush it in order to move on to the next thing.

LINKING THE BREATH TO THOUGHTS AND FEELINGS

- Find a peaceful place and sit or lie down, whichever is more comfortable. Once you are familiar with this exercise you can practise it while standing in a queue, walking, or cooking
- First, breathe in and out
- Observe the wonder of the process. The breath is life. Feel the lungs and body filling up with air and then releasing it. Gently, slowly let go into the natural flow
- To begin with you may need to let out some heavy sighs. You can imagine breathing in light, love, life

• To increase your awareness say to yourself: "When I breathe in, I know I am breathing in" and, "When I breathe out, I know I am breathing out". (This may seem obvious, but breathing has become a totally mechanical and unvalued act.)

• If thoughts come up that distract you, try saying to yourself: "I am thinking this thought, and I'm breathing in" and, "I'm thinking that thought, and I'm breathing out"

• Don't try to escape or suppress your thoughts – this creates more tension and stiffness in the body. Try not to judge any thoughts, such as, "I feel stupid doing this exercise" or, "This is boring". Just bring awareness to your thoughts and to your breathing

• When you notice your thoughts and your feelings, you begin to connect them up with your breathing and accept that they are there. As you continue to observe your breath you are inviting your mind to join up with your body

• As you relax more, so too will your breathing; it will become more harmonious

• We share our air and are deeply interconnected to one another by the breath

• Affirm with each breath, "Yes! I am alive! I receive this life breath and am releasing it with gratitude"

• Breathing awareness restores wholeness, and in this simple exercise you have already begun to heal the body-mind split that leads to ill-health. Awareness of breathing can alleviate many conditions, because when the breath becomes more rhythmical, your general mental and physical health will improve (see also pp. 73-7)

If yin and yang are in perfect balance and flow, and if you continue to be in the present moment, you can achieve a harmonious unity of a mind and body, which becomes a power, a wholeness, and a beauty in itself.

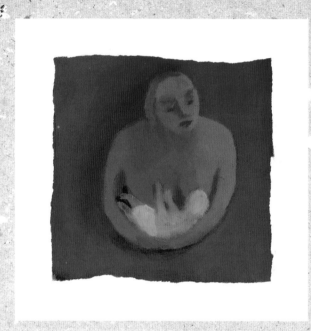

CHAPTER 2

THE FEMALE BODY AND CREATION OF NEW LIFE

*"At a time when few parts of the earth remain
unexplored, in the human body there is still uncharted
territory – and the female body may be the most
mysterious territory of all."*
JOSLEEN WILSON, WOMAN: YOUR BODY, YOUR HEALTH

The Book of Genesis states that in the beginning God created man, and out of Adam's body was created woman.
Implicit in this, and accepted throughout the Judeo-
Christian world, is the establishment of the hierarchy of the
sexes: man first, woman second.

The female body is not a version or adaptation of the
male's, merely created from Adam's spare rib. Women are
whole, healthy, beautiful, and unique. Our seasons coin-
cide with the moon's; our vagina receives the seeds of
future generations; our womb nurtures new life; our
breasts fill with milk to nourish our babies; our curves and
contours reflect the beauty of femininity; we are tall and
short; full and thin; young and old. The yin principle (sym-
bolizing the feminine) stands for creativity and passivity.
But women can also be strong, protective, powerful, and
assertive. We are half the sky.

Men's bodies are whole, healthy, and beautiful, too.
They also have seasons, deeply connected to Nature (see
pp. 104-5); their frame, originally designed for hunting, can
be strong and protective. Men are taller, they run faster,
their sexual organs grow to implant the seeds of new life.

31

Yang stands for outwardness and direct action, but men can also be vulnerable, nurturing, sensitive, and yielding. They are the other half of the sky. The ideal is a meeting of male and female energies, in harmony and balance.

The masculine and feminine exist in both sexes, for how can a man not be feminine when he begins life in his mother's body, and a woman not be masculine when she is partly created by a man? There is no male wholly without feminine characteristics, and no female without masculine attributes. The two completely balanced powers are held together in the all-embracing circle of unity.

Throughout history – and even in today's so-called liberated society – women, their emotions, and their bodies remain, for the most part, misunderstood and misjudged. To understand a woman's body it is important to look at the physiological and spiritual aspects simultaneously, within a holistic framework. Orthodox (conventional) medicine has evolved to view and treat the body as a series of unconnected "bits" and "parts", yet simply possessing a knowledge of the workings of the body does not offer an automatic path to understanding what makes us healthy. Instead of describing the body in terms of organs – heart, lungs, liver, brain, muscles – this book explores the female body in relation to emotions and energies. Your body, nature, and life are deeply connected, and your state of mind can change the state of your body by working through the central nervous system, the endocrine system, and the immune system.

The body's emotions

Everything in Nature is balanced, alive, and in constant motion: and your body is, too. It is a delicately balanced instrument. It is not static or weak, but has strength, movement, and power. The elements that make up your body are like a finely tuned orchestra, and when you are in touch with your feelings, you can conduct your own "orchestra".

Your body is a reflection of who you are. Look at your body and consider the feeling and thinking person that

*One of the reasons we wear lip-
stick is so that our reddened
lips emulate the vagina during
sexual arousal, as a primitive
and unconscious signal to
attract a partner.*

*"After my mastectomy I did
not feel like a real woman. My
breasts seemed to symbolize
everything that was womanly,
beautiful and sexual about
me."*
DOROTHY

lives inside it. Look at the different systems of your body,
just as you contemplate the rivers, mountains, trees,
oceans, and clouds of the Earth. Each is part of the whole.

LOOKING WITHOUT, LOOKING WITHIN
- Create a peaceful space for yourself
- In your mind's eye, visualize yourself naked. Let
your eyes travel down your body, beginning with
your head. Be aware of your breath, thoughts, body,
and feelings at each stage of this exploration
- Imagine breathing in soft, golden light with each
breath, which heals and energizes your body and
internal organs
- Notice your thoughts. If one comes up that distracts you simply acknowledge it and let it be
- Start with your hair, which is often the first thing
women notice in the mirror. You may feel depressed
if your hair does not look healthy. Your hair can be
likened to the "fire" in your body, your aura
- Now visualize your facial features. Ask yourself if
you feel happy about the way you look and try not
to be judgemental. Explore the contours of your face
with your fingers
- Now picture your breasts. They are universal symbols of femininity. Our breasts vary widely in shape
and size, but all variations are normal and do not
affect their function or responsiveness. Move your
hands across your body to caress them
- Picture your pelvic area, where your reproductive
organs lie. Breathe in and out. Gently place your
hands on your pelvic region. Your vulva is not an
organ, but a series of outer folds that protect the
vagina. The outer folds include the outer vaginal
lips, the inner lips, the clitoris, and urethra, as well
as two pairs of lubricating glands
- Now visualize your vagina. This is the connecting
"love channel" between the vulva and internal
organs. Feel the outside. Now gently feel inside. It is

lined with surface tissue similar to the inside of your mouth. It is astonishingly flexible. It guides a penis inside, can stretch and contract around a penis of any size, holds the pools of semen close to the cervix to help conception, acts as a channel for menstrual blood flowing out of your body, and it is a baby's final passageway before birth

• Now imagine your cervix. Insert your finger gently inside your vagina, to feel the tip (similar to the tip of your nose). The cervix is a short, valve-like organ between the vagina and uterus, which allows these two organs to interact. It is about 0.7cm in diameter, if you have not had a baby and up to 3.5cm if you have. In the middle is a very small hole through which sperm enter the uterus and blood flows out during menstruation, and which stretches to allow a baby to pass during birth

• Visualize your uterus (womb). It is pear-shaped and round, soft and muscular to the touch; usually no more than 7cm (three inches) long, during pregnancy it expands considerably. The smooth muscle cells, under the influence of hormones, are constantly in motion, contracting and relaxing throughout the month. During menstruation, as the interior lining is shed, the contractions are strong, and stronger still during childbirth. The womb has a soft inner lining, which is shed every month. If, however, conception occurs and an embryo is implanted in the uterus, this lining becomes a bed for the placenta

• Now move your fingers across your belly and try to visualize the site of the fallopian tubes. They branch out from the upper corners of your womb, leading to the ovaries. They are the vital channels of transport for your eggs, and the place where fertilization occurs. The delicate 10cm (four-inch) tubes are densely lined with cells possessing brush-like tips, which sweep each egg forward into the uterus as it is released. At the top of each fallopian tube,

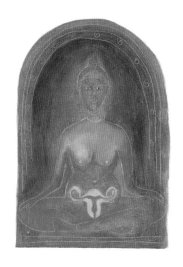

Symbolism and the body
In Russian the word for womb is "matka" meaning "mother". Symbolic of life and fertility, the womb is also sacred and spiritual and the seat of deep emotion and fear.

where it meets the ovary, is a funnel-shaped opening called the fimbria. When an egg that erupts from the surface of the ovary drops on to a petal of the fimbria it is scooped up and swept into the fallopian tube
• Now visualize your ovaries, which, like the testicles, are the primary sexual organs. They develop and release eggs, and pump out the female hormones estrogen and progesterone. After puberty, one egg is released each month. This process is called ovulation (see pp. 80-3)
Your entire female body has potential – for growth, receptivity, expansion, and life. The organs lying within you are in constant motion. Be aware of their rhythms: the constant beat of your heart, the inner ocean of your vaginal secretions, your cycle of ovulation, and the miraculous ebb and flow of minute amounts of hormones.

The mind-body bridge
The breath is the powerful bridge connecting mind to body. Many dis-eases could be avoided were we to develop an awareness of breathing.

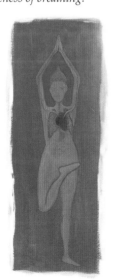

DEVELOPING BODY AWARENESS

Your body expresses your feelings: when you are relaxed, your body feels free and loose; when you are stressed or anxious, it tightens. Your body stiffens to protect itself from both physical and emotional pain. For example, to ward off a blow to the belly your abdominal muscles will automatically tighten. Similarly, if you are upset and cannot give vent to anger or fear, you may suppress your feelings by holding the breath, tensing the throat, and tightening the abdominal muscles. Your body develops these defences for protection against pain and fear. But over time, tensions in your muscles affect your posture, balance, and the flow of energy. Long-term, such imbalances lead to rounded shoulders, distortion of the pelvis, and stiff knees and neck.

The best way to become relaxed is firstly to recognize the stiffness in your body. Do this by practising breathing awareness (see pp. 28-30, 74-7), and noting where the tensions lie. Once you have developed this awareness, you can begin to regain the body's natural elasticity by stretching and practising yoga relaxation exercises.

Becoming familiar with the emotional symbolism of the different parts of your body is another part of awareness. This will help you understand how particular muscle tensions have emotional connections, which may relate to holding in different parts of your personality. If your shoulders feel stiff, perhaps you are feeling overburdened, or continuously over-responsible – you have "too much on your shoulders". Tension around your eyes may reflect the tears you are holding in. Tension in your arms may be an expression of your need to hit, or reach out to others.

You can use these associations to increase your intuition and growing awareness of your body. The following exercise starts the process that begins to bridge the mind-body split, by bringing to light feelings about your body and how you treat it day to day.

"After my lover left me for another woman my womb began to ache, and my period was so heavy I was almost haemorrhaging. I somehow related this to the sudden loss of love which had occurred in my life."
MARIANNE

HOW YOU RELATE TO YOUR BODY
• Put a cushion in front of you and imagine placing your body on it
• Look directly at the cushion, and imagine you are talking to your body. Start by telling it the things you like and dislike about it
• Address your body directly as if it were a person, don't be afraid to say, if it is appropriate, "Body, you're too fat", or, "Your sexuality frightens me". Direct your attention to your thoughts, body, and breathing. If a thought comes up to distract you, simply acknowledge it and let it be. Then continue with the exercise
• After a while, change over, go to sit on the cushion and imagine you are your body speaking back. How would it respond to the things you have told it? Perhaps it might say, "It's you who feeds me when I am not hungry" or, "You don't let me enjoy my sexuality at all!"
• Let your body say what is beautiful about it, and what valuable functions it performs for you
• Then let it say how you could live your life differ-

ently if you listened to its wisdom more. See if there are any demands your body would like to make, such as, "Don't put me in those tight jeans. . .Don't smoke so much. . .Do more meditation. . .Let me get close to another person sexually again"

• After a while, exchange roles again and answer back to your body, letting the dialogue continue

Through language, you have begun to bridge the split between your body and your mind. You may wish to share your discoveries about your relationship with your body with a partner or a friend.

Your subtle energies

How often have you said "I really got a bad feeling from that place", or, "The chemistry between us was great"? Or have you ever walked into a room and just sensed that you didn't want to be there, or alternatively found you could not keep away from a certain person or place? We have an ability to know without knowing. This ability is not recognized by science but we should trust it more – we are sensing subtle energies.

Ancient cultures do recognize these subtle energies, for example, many religions speak of seeing light (an aura) around people's heads. Ancient Indian spiritual tradition speaks of a universal energy called "prana" – the breath of life – which moves through all forms. The Chinese put forward the existence of a vital energy – Ch'i – which contains the two polar forces of yin and yang (see also p. 25).

THE CHAKRAS

The ancient Indian Sanskrit word "Chakra" means circle and movement. Chakras are psychic centres in the body that are active at all times and are central to our health. The chakras work in co-ordination with our nervous system, cells, and fibres. Energy flows the length of our body, along channels and through chakras, to produce different psychic and emotional states. The chakra system is another way of looking at the relationship between the body and the personality, and how we relate to the outside world.

Although it is rare to actually see the chakras, you may regularly feel the sensations without realizing their origin. Chakra sensations include, for example, the feeling of butterflies in your stomach when you are nervous or frightened; tightness in your throat when you want to speak but can't find the words; and the warm, melting sensation in the lower belly when you begin to feel sexually aroused. The middle of the chest, where the heart chakra is found, is a particularly common place to experience sensations. Recall that feeling in your chest when you saw your lover after a long separation – it was from the heart chakra that your love flowed, and it is the heart chakra that produces the pain of heartbreak at the end of an affair.

The first, root, or "base" chakra is located at the base of the spine and in women is located at the vagina. It is associated with sex drive and "grounding". It is connected to the material and physical bases of our lives and our relationship with the material world. It governs the spinal column and kidneys. For women, the root chakra relates particularly to fertility, uterine healing, and to blood and menarche – a girl's first menstruation.

The second chakra is located in the belly and is referred to as our "centre". It is the source of our strength and physical power, vitality, instinctual movement, and sexuality. It governs the reproductive system and is related to issues of pre-orgasm, sexual reopening after painful relationships, ovarian cysts, fertility, menstruation, and menstrual pain.

The third chakra, in the area of the diaphragm and solar plexus, is the seat of raw emotions, anger and fear, and of strong personal attachments. It governs the stomach, liver, gall bladder, and nervous system, and is related to eating disorders, urinary infections, willpower, and visualization.

The fourth, or "heart" chakra, is associated with feelings of compassionate love. It governs the heart, blood, vagus nerve, and circulatory system. Heart chakra issues relate to broken hearts, loneliness, love, self-image, and recovery from childhood abuse or poor relationships.

Eve could do no right
In asserting her natural instinct of curiosity Eve is on record as committing the first sin – eating the forbidden fruit and leading Adam astray. Had she not taken the risk to explore her creativity, the story might have ended there!

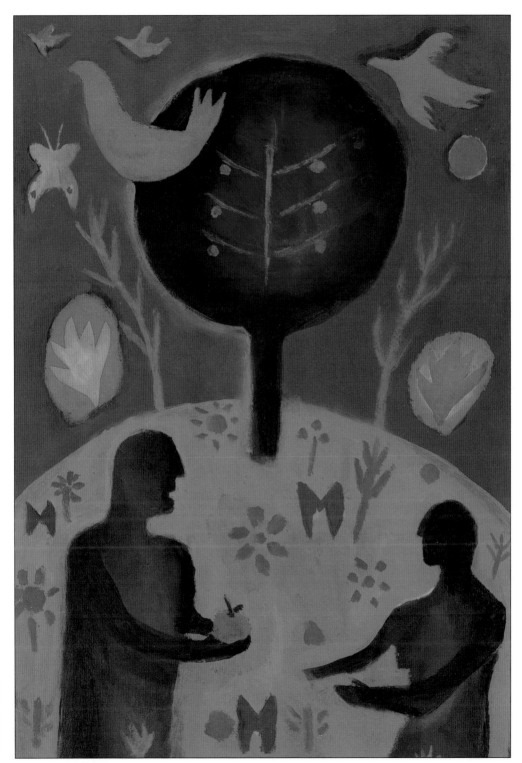

Giovanna Pierce

The fifth centre, in the throat, is linked with self-expression and creativity. It governs the bronchial and vocal apparatus, lungs, and alimentary canal. The throat centre is related to expression, the voice, inflammation, headaches, and rape and incest recovery. Since women are taught to hold in their feelings of anger, pain, and outrage, internalized anger is the cause of most throat-centre healing issues.

The sixth chakra, on the brow, is connected with intellect and intuition, and it governs the lower brain, left eye, ears, nose, and nervous system. Healing uses for this chakra are endocrine balancing, menstrual cycle regulation, the immune system, clairvoyance, and inner healing.

The crown (seventh) chakra at the top and back of the head is linked with spiritual development. It governs the upper brain and right eye and is located where a baby's fontanelle is open at birth, and is the site of women's connection with the goddess. The crown chakra is related to degenerative diseases, stress, white blood cells, tumours, and any issues of the head or brain.

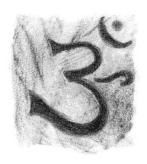

The OM character
This represents the sound released while visualizing the seventh, or crown, chakra, which is linked with spiritual development.

CHAKRAS AND INTIMATE HEALTH

The functions of the chakras are to vitalize the physical body, bring about the development of different aspects of self-awareness, and transmit energy. They are one expression of our spiritual energy body. Illness is caused by an imbalance of energy or a block in the energy flow. This imbalance can also distort your body posture, your perceptions, and inhibit your feelings.

It is important to open the chakras to increase energy flow; the more energy that flows, the healthier you become. For example, if your heart chakra is open and functioning well, your ability to love will be too. When the sixth (intellect) and third (solar plexus) chakras are functioning well, they can enhance your ability to think clearly; however, if they are blocked, your thoughts may be confused.

When two people come together in an intimate relationship, the pattern of activity of one person's chakra connects with that of the partner. You and your partner may link more strongly through some chakras than others. These differences are expressed in the comments people make about their relationship – that, for example, it is "primarily sexual", or "a strong spiritual bond". The inexplicable chakra bond explains why it can be so painful to separate from a relationship. Sometimes you may carry another person's energy in your field and need consciously to release it to allow in new, healthier relationships.

As a woman matures and develops, each chakra represents the psychological patterns evolving in her life. Just as your body has a natural "armour" to protect itself from attack, you may react defensively to painful experiences by blocking your feelings. This restricts a great deal of your natural energy flow. If, for example, as a child, you were rejected or abused every time you tried to express love, you will probably stop trying to love. When this occurs the energy flow through the heart chakra is blocked.

When a chakra is blocked, a physical problem is likely to result. For example, suppressed or unexpressed rage may result in pelvic infections, because you are blocking powerful sexual feelings by holding them tightly in your pelvis. The accumulation of stagnated energy in your pelvis can bring about conditions such as pelvic inflammatory disease or endometriosis.

If you experience these or other conditions, try not to judge yourself harshly. Instead, gently find out the meaning and healing required. It is always a long process and do not be discouraged if it takes longer than you had thought. Body changes can be slower than the mind.

THE AURA

Where conventional medicine treats the physical symptoms only, chakra-healing works with the body through unseen psychic layers.

The body is surrounded by an electrical field, called the "aura". This is composed of four unseen bodies that surround and affect the physical body. In esoteric thought, the aura is where our soul or "being" is located, and it also directs the physical body's health and growth.

The first of the four bodies is called the "physical body"

The sounds and colour of chakras
When visualizing a chakra, it may help if you release a sound and picture coloured light radiating out from the centre. Each chakra has its own associated colour and sound.
The first chakra is red and its sound is OOO (as in "you")
The second chakra is orange in colour and its sound is OH (as in "home")
The third chakra is yellow and its associated sound is AW (as in "saw")
The fourth chakra is green and its vibrating sound is AAH (as in "far")
The fifth chakra is blue in colour and its sound is EH (as in "egg")
The sixth chakra has an indigo colour and its vibrating sound is EEE (as in "bee")
The seventh chakra is violet-white in colour and its sound is OM (as in "from")

or "etheric double" aura. It is the vibrating light that surrounds and follows the body's contours. Illness appears
first at this level, and the seven chakras are located on the
physical body aura.

Moving outward from the skin, next to the physical
body aura, is the "emotional body". This energy layer gen-
erates and transmits emotions, through the etheric to the
physical body. Emotions are important, since unreleased
feelings can turn inward to cause physical illness. Clearing
the body of held-in pain and fear, to release blocked emotions, is a major part of women's healing. Emotions can be
locked in the physical body: to allow them to flow again, a
balance is required. You need to release your locked emotions before you can let in the new. Conscious breathing
will help move the emotions and bring back a healthy flow.
The emotional body is dynamic, constantly fluctuating and
moving. When flowing, it expands beyond your physical
body and when you feel open and expansive your emotional body is larger and even further out from the body.

The third of the aura bodies is the "mental body", which
contains the rational and imaginative mind. The mind and
imagination are important tools, which can generate either
health or dis-ease. You may actually be able to create what
you think, and what you imagine may become real. You
have the power to make negative images happen and you
also have the power to transmit positive images telling
your physical body what to do.

The fourth unseen body is the "spiritual body". The
more closely you accept yourself as part of Nature, the
more healing power you are able to transmit through this
spiritual body to all the other layers.

ENERGY AS MEDICINE

Some people can see, or sense the chakras as coloured light
or energy radiating from the body at different points. Some
health practitioners use the chakra map to gain an overall
view of a woman's life and personality.

Certain clairvoyants are able to see or feel the chakras
through their hands. They are able to identify illnesses and

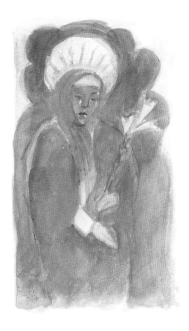

The halo – what is it?
In religious art Christ and
other saints and spiritual
figures are often portrayed
surrounded by circles of light
or halos. The halo symbolizes
the energy layers or "aura",
that surround the body.

blocked channels in people before they are manifest in the body, which suggests that the dysfunction appears in the energy field first, and then shows up in the body.

The auras are where your thoughts, emotions, and your being reside. Your body merely reflects what is happening in your energy field. The flow of energy through each chakra reflects how open or blocked you are in each of these areas of your life.

When working with the chakras, the emphasis is on balance. The aim is to achieve a harmonious relationship between the different chakras and the aspects they govern – physical, sexual, emotional, intuitive, intellectual, and spiritual. For example, if a woman is underdeveloped in her "root" chakra (see p. 38) she might be helped by leg and foot massage, or breathing mindfulness (see pp. 28-30) that focuses on that part of her body, or by encouragement to explore her feelings about her sexuality.

Some alternative therapists, such as acupuncturists and homeopaths, will try to detect areas of weakness and potential dysfunction in your body. They will endeavour to strengthen your body's vital force or "chi" back to health.

Chakra healing usually involves laying-on of hands, massage, and helping you become aware of suppressed emotional conflicts. In time you will develop more mature thinking processes, and find new solutions to old problems, inappropriate coping mechanisms, and out-of-date thought patterns.

Even people who cannot see an aura or energy field around a person's body, may be able to sense it with their hands. To gain a clearer understanding of how chakras can help you get more in touch with your body, and therefore improve your health, try the following three exercises.

SENSING THE CHAKRAS

The first step toward exploring the chakras for yourself is simply to relax, send your awareness to the site of each chakra in turn, and notice what you experience. You may draw a blank, or you may

---

The chakra bond

Psychics seeing two people together can sometimes perceive the connections between them, and tell which chakras are strong and which need to be strengthened, in order to create a more balanced relationship.

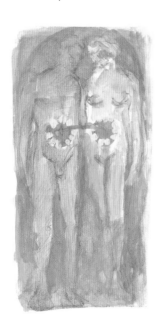

come up with images or thoughts that increase your self-understanding.

• Sit or lie comfortably with arms and knees uncrossed. Relax for a few minutes, just noticing your breathing

• Now send your awareness to your root chakra. Place your fingers on the point of the chakra to help you make contact. Notice any sensations, symbols, thoughts, or associations that arise. Imagine the colour red here

• Continue for ten minutes

• Afterward write down or tell a friend what came up for you

• Repeat this exercise for each of the other chakras (see pp. 38-41 for the exact chakra positions and their corresponding colours and sounds)

SENSING AN ENERGY FIELD

• Sit opposite your partner, with your palms touching. Let the energy flow naturally. Sense the pulsating flow for a while. Which way does it go?

• Send energy out of your left palm; then allow it to come into your right. Reverse. Now stop the flow

• Next try pushing it out of both hands at once. Now draw it in to both hands at once. Push, pull, and stop are three basic ways to manipulate energy in healing

• Now, drop hands. Hold your palms 5-12cm (two to five inches) apart; slowly move your hands back and forth decreasing and increasing the space between them. A warm sensation begins to generate between your hands. What does it feel like?

• Now, take your hands further apart, 20-25cm (eight to ten inches), and slowly bring them back together until you feel a pressure pushing your hands out so that you have to use a slightly stronger force to bring your hands together

• Now, take your hands apart again and hold them at a distance of about 18cm (seven inches). Point your right index finger at the palm of your left hand, making sure the fingertip is about 1-3cm (one half to one inch) away from the palm. Now, draw circles on your palms. What do you feel? Does it tickle?

SENSING A PERSON'S ENERGY

Phrases such as "You're invading my personal space" describe how our psychic space can feel threatened. This exercise will help you to sense the safe zones in which we live and house our beings

• Begin to tune in to the spaces that you regularly visit. Walk into your parents' or a friend's home. How do you feel? Do you like it? Do you want to stay, or do you want to leave?

• If you have children, go into each of their rooms. Feel the difference in the energy in each room. How does it match your child? What aspects of him or her does it express?

• Is the decor and colour right for them, or is it one you have imposed on their space? Think about it

• Try this exercise with different places that you go into, and you will notice how you may find it impossible to stay in certain places because of the energy emanating there, but feel drawn to others. The more in touch you are with your inner being, the more powerfully you will be able to go toward things, people, and places that support you in your life

Our beginnings

Some women say they can "psychically sense" the moment of conception, but for others this deeply private moment will vary greatly in terms of awareness and experience .

With recent advances in foetal diagnosis and therapy, researchers are constantly piecing together new information on the unborn child. Much of the child's physical behaviour can now be observed in utero – inside the womb before birth – which enables us to revisit that stage of our life, which none of us can consciously recall.

LIFE INSIDE YOUR MOTHER'S BODY

To become more in touch with yourself, it is helpful to imagine your wondrous journey in your mother's body. Biologically, your life began when one survivor out of thousands of sperm penetrated your mother's egg, lying within the fallopian tube. The egg is genetically female (X); your sex was determined by your father's sperm – which can carry a male (Y) or a female (X) chromosome. The balance of yin and yang (see p. 25) is present at the very beginnings of life.

At two weeks you had, in primitive form, both male and female parts. By the fifth week you had developed ovaries and had begun to form fallopian tubes and a vagina. Here lie the origins of your femaleness.

THE EMOTIONAL DEVELOPMENT OF YOUR UNBORN BABY

We cannot alter or predict specific personality traits, nor should we want to, but a new awareness of the unborn baby as a thinking, feeling, creative person can make a difference. It can help us to identify and prevent the beginnings of both physical and psychological problems.

The womb was our first home. How we experienced it – as loving, hostile, or balanced – shaped our personality and emotional predispositions.

The Chinese consider pregnancy to be a yin state for the mother, who must concentrate on her environment within, and a yang state for the unborn baby. During pregnancy, the mother, influenced by her increased hormones, usually becomes more yin, sensitive, and emotional. A pregnant woman needs constant support, shelter, and love from her partner. Excessive yang (outgoing and active) activities for a pregnant woman can create imbalance and lead to a difficult birth, and problems for the baby.

The Chinese established the first prenatal clinics one thousand years ago. They were well aware that a mother's experiences impressed themselves on her unborn child. What unborn babies feel and perceive in the womb begins shaping their attitudes and expectations about themselves. If the womb environment is loving and warm, your baby is

"We made intense love, having made a conscious decision to have a child, and I knew immediately the moment I had conceived. I lay in my partner's arms, and felt at once elated, scared, happy, and apprehensive."
KATY

46

likely to expect the outside world to be the same, and receive a sense of trust, openness, and self-confidence. If the womb environment has been hostile, your baby might anticipate that the new world will be equally uninviting.

The ill-effects of poor diet, drinking, and drug-taking during pregnancy are well-documented. Less studied is that your emotions, thoughts, and feelings may be communicated to and have influence on your unborn child. Your thoughts and feelings are just one element among many that shape your unborn baby's emotional development. What makes them a unique element is that, unlike genetic inheritance, they are controllable. Through increased awareness you can make them a positive force, and use them to affect your baby's development for the good.

YIN-YANG AS MOTHER-FATHER

We are created out of a union of a woman and a man: yin and yang. That magical and harmonious combination remains a vital factor throughout our entire life for our growth and emotional development, as well as our physical, sexual, and spiritual health.

The love and presence of your baby's father is needed to introduce the yang (outer) world to your child. In this sense the male/female balance of yin-yang is essential to your child during pregnancy and birth, and particularly during early life. The quality of the parents' relationship can influence the infant's development. According to studies carried out in Austria and Germany, a poor relationship between the parents can be among the greatest causes of emotional and physical damage to the unborn child. However a strong, nurturing mother-child emotional bond during pregnancy (intra-uterine bonding) can protect your unborn baby against even severe trauma.

COMMUNICATING WITH BABY IN THE WOMB

In ancient China and Japan, as well as maintaining a lifestyle conducive to their child's emotional wellbeing, pregnant women were encouraged to spend time communicating with their babies in the womb each day. This practice – known as tai-kyo – was based on the principle that your health and happiness can affect your baby, both physically and emotionally.

The best period for intra-uterine bonding is the last three months of pregnancy, particularly the last two, when the baby is mature enough physically and emotionally to send and receive fairly sophisticated messages. As the mother, you set the pace, provide the cues, and mould your baby's responses. If your moves are contradictory or hostile your baby may ignore them or become confused, so an understanding of your own feelings is needed to make the bonding happen. If you shut down emotionally, and therefore feel cut off from your feelings, your baby is at a loss. Sensitive counselling during pregnancy might be helpful, and may even prevent post-natal depression.

Even if a trauma occurs during pregnancy, your baby need not suffer, and will continue to thrive, so long as you keep the channels of communication between yourself and your child open and flowing with reassuring messages. At the moment of conception you entered into a relationship with your unborn baby. By becoming more conscious and aware of the way you and your baby can communicate, you can nurture your relationship.

HOW TO ENHANCE THE RELATIONSHIP WITH YOUR UNBORN BABY

• Communicate by talking, meditating, and deep breathing. Focus your attention inward (yin) to connect with your baby. Reassure your baby that s/he is safe in your body; is loved and wanted. A soft, soothing tone of voice will reinforce this

• Spend a few minutes each day relaxing by listening to soothing music, practising gentle yoga postures, or being sensuously bathed and massaged by your partner. If you feel relaxed, secure, and tranquil, so will your baby. Your baby will enjoy and respond to chanting, singing, and instrumental music. Your baby will also benefit from your rhythmic body-movements when you exercise,

dance, swim, or make love
• Kicking is your unborn baby's most easily
measured form of communication. Any number of
things may provoke it, from anxiety, excitement, and
joy to fear and anger. By kicking, your baby is also
discovering movement, boundaries, and the uterine
wall, and may even be reacting to loud music

The most natural way to communicate physically
with your baby is to rub your abdomen, a gesture of
reassurance, which is universal among pregnant
women and is almost subconscious
• Spiritual communication is a form of intuitive
knowledge, a sensing of your baby's needs. The
more you are in touch with your own "inner child" –
the child you once were – the more sensitive you will
be to the baby developing in your womb
• Dreams during pregnancy – which are often vivid
and strange – can express both wishes and unconscious conflicts about your child. This is one of the
beneficial ways pregnant women deal with their
anxieties. Dreams may also be an extrasensory communication from your child, through which s/he
tries to convey a message to you
• Take particular care to avoid smoking, excessive
drinking, and drug-taking during pregnancy, and
eat a balanced diet
• Rest assured that not everything you do, such as
having an occasional negative thought, is going to
affect your relationship with your child. The danger
only arises when your baby feels shut off from you,
or when the baby's physical and psychological
needs are consistently ignored

MEDITATION AND AWARENESS DURING PREGNANCY
This meditation exercise will help you to communicate with your unborn child. Meditating in this way
for a few minutes every day, and just being with
your baby, will help you to retain an inner sense of

your child's presence. Even if your day has been difficult and tiring, as it often is for many women during pregnancy, these few moments will give you the opportunity consciously to communicate loving messages to your baby and your "inner child".

• Sit comfortably with your eyes closed. Breathe deeply and relax, allowing yourself to become quiet, calm, and centred. Repeat the exercise on mindfulness of breathing (see pp. 28-30)

• Focus inwardly on the presence of your baby

• Place your hands over your belly and gently caress it. Feel the warmth and tingling in your hands

• Feel your baby's gentle movements within

• Take your time, visualize your baby's tiny body inside your womb – head, arms, legs, hands, feet, fingers, and toes

• Really try and visualize your baby. What does s/he look like? What impressions do you get?

• What kind of a mover is s/he – slow, or quick? (Impressions may be accurate or totally inaccurate. It does not matter.)

• Imagine how the warm amniotic fluid must feel on the sensitive surface of your baby's skin, and what it must be like to move and somersault at will

• Ask your baby what music s/he enjoys. Generally babies prefer gentle, soothing, rippling sounds, although some babies enjoy more dynamic music

• Imagine the sounds that your baby hears – your voice, the reassuring regularity of your heartbeat, and the rumblings of your digestive system. S/he may also be hearing music, the father's voice, and other sounds from outside the womb

• Close to the birth, ask your baby what he or she is experiencing. Reassure your baby not to worry about the space shortage. You both know the birth time is drawing near

Nurture
An infant's instincts lead the child to "use" the mother for nurture. If the mother can withstand this willingly, and "hold", or contain, the child's feelings, the baby's selfhood is more assured, and the mother is less likely to feel she is "being used", which can make her feel anonymous.

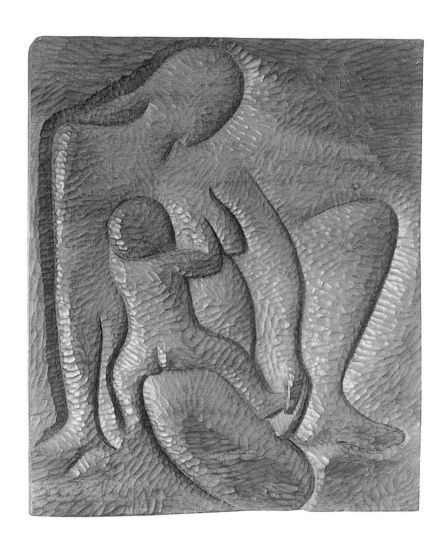

The birth experience

"The baby knows everything. Feels everything. The baby sees right into our hearts, knows the colour of our thoughts. All without language. The newborn baby is a mirror, reflecting our image. It is up to us to see it doesn't cry." Frederick Leboyer, *Birth Without Violence*

Birth is a momentous time for a baby, but it is probably even more momentous for the mother. Some women feel that it is the most significant and spiritual event they have ever experienced. Perhaps this is because it is a time of reckoning, when life is in balance, and when a woman is brought into contact with her own mortality for the first time. Birth is also an important time for the couple as a unit. A woman giving birth needs her partner with her not only for support, but also to share in the spiritual arrival of the baby. The couple may feel deep love passing between them, which they can then transmit to the baby. The father may be able to feel a sense of his own importance in the family. He will more easily "believe" the birth "miracle" and feel highly valued right from the start of his child's life. This may help him to bond from the very moment of birth and develop a close relationship in the years ahead with his child.

The midwife is waiting patiently in the fifteenth hour of a labour that is progressing well. She is in touch with – and attuned to – the mother's natural rhythms, and because she is working from a feminine principle, she does not interfere. Enter the obstetrician, who, because of his/her training, is working more from a masculine (active) principle and therefore has the urge to control or intervene. Only if the baby or mother is in distress will the masculine principle of intervention be wholly appropriate. The best outcome will follow a balanced approach, and, as attitudes gradually shift, midwives and obstetricians now have more mutual respect and will to work in harmony than ever before. It is possible to be helped through even the most "difficult birth" (where the use of high-tech equipment and drugs is crucial), yet still draw on natural birthing techniques to uphold the spirituality of the event. A midwife working to the feminine principle can coexist with an obstetrician working to the masculine principle because each can complement the other. But the will to do so must be there in the first place.

Our memories of birth are held in every cell of our bodies, and can affect our whole mental, emotional, physical, sexual, and spiritual wellbeing. The quality of birth can affect the quality of life, which in turn shapes the quality of society as a whole.

More than any other aspect of women's health care, pregnancy and birthing practices have undergone tremendous changes. These changes began with birth pioneer Frederick Leboyer, and were further developed by groundbreaking books such as *Immaculate Deception* (1975) by Suzanne Arms and organizations such as the British National Childbirth Trust and the Home Birth Movement. All recognized the dominance of the masculine in obstetrics, and helped to open the way to allowing women to follow and have trust in the natural instinct and feminine wisdom of their bodies: to give birth in their own way, with support rather than interference.

Some women are now choosing the water-birth method. They float in a pool of deep, warm water during labour, and can also deliver the baby there, if they wish. Obstetricians who value such methods are likely to be in touch with, attuned to, and in balance with their own masculine and feminine sides. They will allow and encourage this in their patients and midwives.

The approach to birth that respects and honours a woman's wisdom, natural bodily functions, and the sacredness of birth, upholds the suggestions I am making to improve women's intimate health care: that it is important to encourage a woman to make contact with the deeper, feminine, instinctual forces within her.

A birth where many medical interventions are required can still be loving, if the people present and the mother especially are tuned in to the holiness of the moment and

Tip for partners and birth attenders
It is tempting to think that a woman giving birth is somehow mentally "somewhere else", and unable to hear or take in things that are said in the delivery room. Remember to be sensitive to her all the time, which includes not talking across her as though she cannot hear you.

relate to the baby with love. It is possible to over-empha-size the actual birth. One can create a water birth, yet not be truly aware of the baby's spirit in presence with love. If we focus more on the mother's drama and the "gallant obste-trician", without due respect for the baby, it is a form of neglect to the baby.

Spirituality is not a separate part of us: it is bound up with the body and the whole person, long before we enter this world. The word "spiritual" is often off-putting or mis-understood, because it is thought to be something esoteric and hard to define. But it is not, it is about coming from your heart!

The physiological aspects of conception, pregnancy, and birth are well documented in myriad pregnancy and birth books, yet the spiritual dimension is rarely acknowledged. Birth is the transition of a soul to earthly life. Love, compas-sion, and spiritual vision are the most important tools of the midwife's, the obstetrician's, and the doctor's trade.

THE QUALITY OF BIRTH AFFECTS FUTURE HEALTH

Birth is a metaphor for all creative processes. Birthing pio-neer Binnie Dansby specializes in rebirthing, that is helping people heal their own birth traumas (see pp. 75-6). Binnie believes that we can transform the quality of lives by improving the quality of the birth experience. She has found that a pregnant woman will often unconsciously recreate her own birth – or sometimes recreate her partner's birth. She helps expectant mothers heal their own births, enabling them to give birth consciously and ecstatically.

A baby who is born surrounded by people who respect, love, and listen to him/her, enters this world with her/his body, mind, and spirit intact. This is the best foundation for a healthy and whole human being.

HOW TO BRING THE FEMININE PRINCIPLE OF "BEING" INTO YOUR BABY'S EARLY LIFE

Through a positive birth experience, a baby learns that the mother's body is healthy, wise, and whole. A gentle transi-tion from womb to the outside world, including if possible

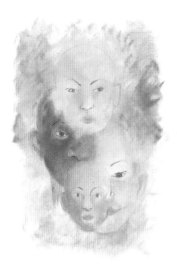

The vital urge
Inside every child is an innate
drive toward growth,
wholeness, and vitality.
Families are crucial in either
fostering or interfering with
this vital impulse.

holding the baby straight away, will give your baby a secure start in life. However, many babies will not be fortunate enough to experience birth in this way. A multitude of reasons may make a caesarean, forceps, and/or various drugs necessary to avoid risking the safety of mother and child. If you prepare yourself for a peaceful, natural birth, but have to go through necessary intervention, you may feel guilty, or somehow a failure. Talk through your feelings with your partner, family, midwife, health visitor, and friends and feel held and supported by their love and sympathy. Through this you will gain confidence that you can give your baby the extra comfort s/he needs. A baby who seems very unsettled after a difficult birth will soon calm, given loving care and attention.

After separation, when the umbilical cord has been cut, maintain physical contact by placing your baby on your stomach, in your arms, or wherever feels comfortable for you both. Your baby needs as much bodily contact as possible. After a caesarean these processes may be delayed, but can still apply, or your baby can be handed to the father, who will be able to welcome his child into the world with warm loving hands and sensitivity. Only gradually, over the next few weeks, will your baby begin to discover separateness from you. Keeping constant physical contact with your baby may seem a tall order, particularly if you have other children demanding your time and attention. Also your partner may find it difficult to accept, consciously or subconsciously, that he has less of your attention. The more you and your partner communicate, express feelings, and support each other, the more you will be able to pass this on to your children.

This early stage, where your baby is unable to differentiate between you and her/himself, may be experienced by you in a similar way. You may feel preoccupied with your infant, as though the child is an extension of yourself; this bond can be very intense in the first weeks after birth.

Initially your baby expects an immediate response to every need, because in the womb everything was continuously supplied through your placenta. Your baby is not used to experiencing feelings of hunger, thirst, and cold. If you do not respond immediately your baby may become anxious, having no understanding that you eventually will respond. Your newborn will not understand that you are "not far away", and will only achieve greater security through your presence and constant responses. You are not "spoiling" by being over-attentive. Your yin ability to empathize and "be", ensures that the unity, which began in your womb, is continued until your baby develops a memory of your reliability and an inner feeling of safety. These adjustments take place in a very short space of time; the transition will occur smoothly if you have a home environment that sensitively provides you with a chance to form a relationship with your baby in an undisturbed and unhurried way.

Gradually, your baby will gain a sense of you as a person. As you speak your baby will "remember" hearing your voice from inside your womb and this, coupled with recognizing your smell, enables your baby to gain a sense of you as a person.

In the womb your baby may have put thumb to mouth, when s/he had the impulse to suck. Your baby expects what has occurred in the womb to continue after birth, with your nipple. Do not pressurize your baby to suck straight away by forcing your nipple into the mouth. When ready your baby will let you know. A baby has enough nutrients and fluids for two to three days after birth, although babies usually begin feeding a day or so after birth. In the very beginning, when your baby seeks your nipple and you respond, the baby thinks that s/he alone has caused your nipple to appear. Your baby wants it, and it magically appears. The beginnings of self-confidence and creativity originate in allowing your infant to feed spontaneously, in response to the impulse to do so.

Caring for your child to help him or her grow into a healthy, integrated being is not following a series of instructions, but rather giving love, awareness, and understanding. If you yourself are in turn supported, encouraged, and allowed to become confident by all those around you, you will more easily allow the development, which takes place naturally in a child, to progress undisturbed. Support for the mother is essential, because the more a mother is in touch with herself and her own feelings, the more she will instinctively know what to do for her child.

It may be a relief to know, however, that your child does not depend entirely upon you for growth and development. Babies are born with a vital urge toward life and maturity, carried forward in ways we may never fully understand. It is like the bulbs we plant in the garden: we know we cannot make them grow into flowers, yet with the right kind of soil, water, and care growth occurs naturally, because the bulbs have life inside them.

Caring for your baby is more complex, but as with the bulbs, inside your child there is a movement toward health, wholeness, and harmony, which with love and mindfulness, you and your partner can help facilitate.

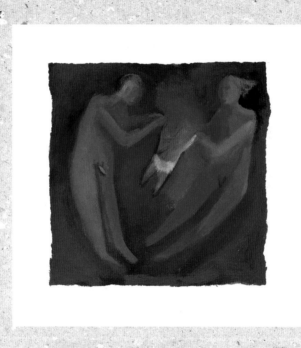

CHAPTER 3

THE EMOTIONS AND WELLBEING

*"It is the capacity for feeling deeply for one another
that binds us together, man to woman, parent to child, friend
to friend. Our emotional nature enables us to experience
compassion for other living beings and to translate this
feeling into positive action."*
NAOMI HUMPHREY, *MEDITATION: THE INNER WAY*

What causes us to feel intensely, and react in certain ways?
What influences us to feel so many different emotions: to
feel hopeless, frightened, happy, angry, or bursting with
joy and love?

Our psyche – like the air we breathe – literally "takes in"
the emotional environment of our early life. How we are
responded to, and then experience, express, and process
our emotions will play a vital role in our future mental and
physical wellbeing. Our ability to cope with, and express
negative emotions such as pain and anger, stems from how
safe and contained our early environment was.

One of the greatest responsibilities of a parent is to create and sustain a loving and welcoming emotional
environment for their children, to enable them to develop
as loving, compassionate, sensitive, and responsible human
beings. Yet it is a task for which we receive little training,
apart from adopting the values we inherit from our own
parental and cultural environment. At best we tend to
muddle through and perhaps, for many people, learning as
we go and relying on our own initiative is as good a way as
any to go about it.

Emotional development

Our emotional development begins as early as the first weeks in our mother's womb. In the 1950s, psychoanalyst Dr Donald Winnicott emphasized the mother-infant relationship, and its importance for an infant's developing emotions. Winnicott coined the phrase a "good enough" mother, stressing that it is impossible to be a perfect parent, or to ensure a perfect childhood. What he did claim is that it is possible for "ordinary" parents – people who are relatively undamaged – to create a "good enough" environment in which their child can grow and develop healthily and happily.

RESTORING THE BALANCE IN PARENTING

Good parenting requires a balance of yin-yang energies according to the varying stages of childhood. In the beginning, after the baby's birth, a mother is in a yin state of simply "being" with her baby at the breast. Yin is required because children need waiting for, not hurrying. Though necessary, this yin time can be taxing on the mother's patience. The yang state is also required, for the mother securely to contain (see p. 62) her baby's emotions. Babies need to have their feelings held, not judged; contained, not driven. However, a predominance of yang during childhood, oriented to goals and efficiency, can make the development process difficult for a child.

An important part of the father's function in a child's early infancy is to foster the union between mother and child: a task he will enjoy if he is comfortable with his feminine side, but avoid and resent if he feels insecure, unfulfilled, and excluded, – unfortunately all too common.

Being aware and in touch with your inner male is important in your role of mother. Indeed, your masculine side can function as an inner husband: strong and loving to protect you and your child from harm and intrusions. Both parents need the space to develop both their masculine and feminine sides, so that the child's vision of the world is not split and stereotyped. This leads to healthier separation as your child grows and develops.

INTIMACY IS YOUR BABY'S FIRST FOOD

How you respond to your baby is crucial, because s/he will experience upset, frustration, and joy in relation to you. A mother's responses affect the developing psyches (personalities) of her children, which explains why the inner image of mother is extremely powerful, and can take on almost magical proportions.

Throughout your child's early years, just as during pregnancy and birth, you need to be consistent in your love and responses. All the processes that begin before birth need to continue thereafter, appropriate to your child's stage of development and unique personality.

The food for your baby's developing personality is primarily human contact. Young babies do not have any sense of self. Your baby may perceive your breast as an extension of her/himself and may not yet recognize boundaries. You can try to bring boundaries into the relationship by relating to your baby as separate from you. Set limits of safety and support for your baby, to provide a sense of containment, which is vital for healthy emotional development.

Your baby's personality will develop naturally through your continued responses, and gradually s/he will be able to maintain a sense of self, even when you are not present. Your baby will embody – take inside her/himself – your love and care, which helps your baby to become secure in the knowledge that you will return. Consistent love, nurturing, and the setting of boundaries will create a sense of psychological wellbeing, which will help to give your child a secure sense of self, self-love, and safety. Parents should discuss and agree on boundaries together, so that they are always consistent and do not have to disagree in front of the child, making her/him feel insecure.

PROJECTION

Infants and children, until they become more resilient, will rely upon having a mother and father who can understand and empathize with their feelings. Since a baby's personality is not mature enough to cope with even minor incidents, a child will push feelings of pain and anger on to the mother, hoping that she will give back love and warmth to take away the pain. This process is called "projection", whereby we put unwanted parts of ourselves into others, and take bits of others back into ourselves. This is how we begin to learn the process of intercourse – giving out and taking in. We simply need to know that our feelings and expressions are safe, manageable, and loveable.

During infancy the mother needs to be the "container" for some of her baby's more intolerable feelings. If the bond between the mother and baby has been disturbed (because of the mother's conflicts, or because she herself has not received adequate love and support), then the baby may experience difficulty in expecting her/his emotions to be acknowledged and contained in future relationships.

To contain, or hold, your baby's feelings, it is best not to retaliate at her/his upset. Let your baby know that whatever s/he feels is fine and that s/he is surrounded by love. To do this you need to feel loved and supported by those around you, especially your partner.

You should try not to suppress your baby's upset, or make light of it or respond to it by shouting or smacking. Try to bear your child's panic, and in doing so, you will show your child that you can survive. Your child will be able to come through these difficult experiences simply because you are able to "hold" the pain and confusion. This in turn will help you feel strong and confident, and better able to cope with the child who can be an expert at challenging her/his parents intolerably.

INDIVIDUATION

As your baby's sense of you and others develops, you will be able to let go to some degree, as s/he gradually begins to separate and become her/his own person. This process is referred to by psychotherapists as "individuation", but in our terms it is the time when your child is establishing a clearer sense of self and independence.

As babies move toward being emotionally separate they learn that people fall into two categories: female and male. By approximately one year old your baby will already be

A bond for life
In the past fathers have felt marginalized: they were not allowed to be present at the birth and often had very little involvement in their child's upbringing. Gradually this is changing; being present at the birth will help the father believe in the birth "miracle" and help him to bond immediately with the baby. By participating fully in all aspects of childcare, the father can nurture this bond, which should then last for life.

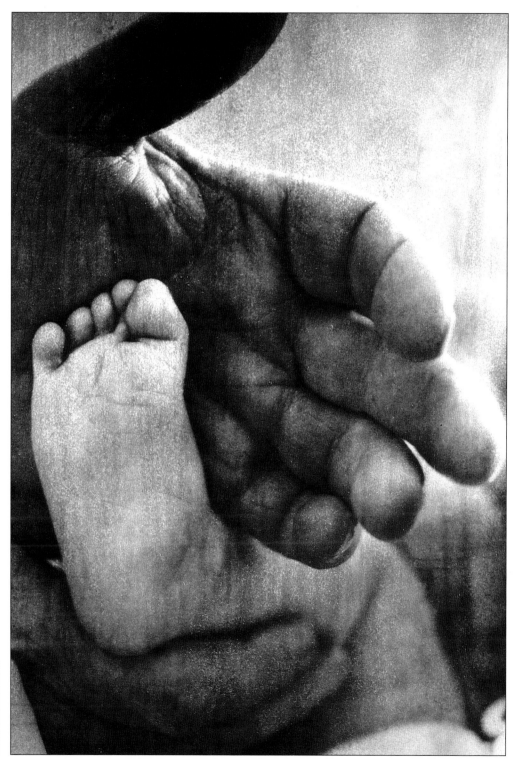

Andreas Heumann

able to recognize and point to men and women as either the mother or father. However, all these stages vary greatly and it is important to remember that every child is unique, growing at an individual pace.

A baby's family will assign a place and role in the world for their child largely based upon gender. In every culture feminine and masculine have different primary behavioural roles. Family members, in relating to a boy, will tend to have different expectations of him than of a girl. Against this complex backdrop is set our development as a woman.

THE MAKING OF A WOMAN

A woman's psychological makeup is a result of a complex combination of influences – parental, peer, family, and the wider social environment – together with the values of the culture in which she is brought up. As we mature, we inevitably also take on board those emotions and behaviour patterns that are considered acceptably "feminine", and "masculine" within that culture.

A girl's psychology develops within the context of the relationship she has with her mother or caregiver, and although the ideal parenting should be a balance between mother and father, it is still the norm for the mother to be the central person at the start of life.

Women generally relate differently to a daughter than to a son. Some of the differences come from unconscious feelings about being a woman, but most importantly, women learn from their mothers about their place in the world. In each woman's experience is the memory, buried or alive, of the struggles she had with her own mother in the process of becoming a woman.

When a woman bears a son, his different gender helps her become more aware of her own boundaries, but with a daughter the boundaries are often blurred. You don't only identify with your daughter, but also project on to her some of the feelings you have about yourself, and experience them as if your daughter is expressing them. You may see her not as another person, but as an extension of yourself: a vulnerable, undefended little girl. This unconsciously awakens that part of you that feels unresponded to and needy.

As a mother, you identify with your daughter because when you give birth to a girl you are, in a sense, reproducing yourself. You may feel that you are your baby, and that the baby is you. Your son is different: he is something else "out there", somebody different. You can imagine for him a world of yang (male) possibilities, but deep down you know your daughter will follow in your yin footsteps.

However, this is by no means always the case. Some mothers have reported that regardless of gender difference, a son can sometimes seem more like themselves than a same-sex child.

As a girl grows up she forms a future image of herself as a woman through the women around her – mother, grandma, aunts, sisters, friends, movie stars, and the media. Sexual stereotypes surround children from the moment of their birth, which means a different psychology is transmitted to girls than to boys. In the West boys are raised expecting to be looked after and attended to, and girls are expected to provide the nurturing. The on-going effect of having to suppress their wants and desires leaves many girls and women unaware of their feelings of neediness. A woman often feels that nobody is aware of her needs, compounded by the fact that even she cannot put her finger on, and express, what she really wants.

A new feminist psychology of women has become essential to the understanding of women's emotional health, since studies suggest that there are cultural and social forces at work in the West that make women more susceptible than men to conditions such as anorexia nervosa, phobias, and psychosomatic disorders.

THE MAKING OF A MAN

Girls, traditionally raised by a woman (the mother), identify with her for the rest of their lives. Boys, however, do not. While both male and female babies identify with mother, internalizing her basic qualities, by the time a boy is eighteen months old he already knows he is male and different

65

from mother. He learns from his father, other males, and from the outside world that being a man means working outside the home, being strong and tough, not crying, and being willing to fight. He learns that men appear to be more dominant and important, that they "run the world".

While the feminine world of the mother is the centre of his universe, a boy knows that in order to become a man he must distance himself from it, separate himself from the less powerful world of women and find his place in the world of men. To do this he represses early feelings of attachment, dependency, vulnerability, and intense love and hate, and represses his desire for the gentler world of women he has grown up in, which is feminine and unfit for "real" men.

Many fathers act in an overly macho fashion with their infant sons, tossing them and throwing them about, in an attempt, conscious or unconscious, "to make them tough", an attitude which polarizes the sex differences even further. A loving, caring, and supportive father, strong yet tender, who does not condone violence, is more likely to have a non-violent son. For such a boy, the separation from the feminine is less defined and more balanced. He can identify with his father and still retain some loving, gentle, empathic qualities.

The division of the sexes into polarized roles can lead to a conflict identity in some boys, especially those without male role models. They may develop an unconscious fear of being feminine, which leads to "protest masculinity" – which can lead on to male "solidarity", even misogyny. According to Myriam Miedzian in *Boys will be Boys* (1992), the more exclusively a boy is reared by women without the presence of a reliable male figure, the more he will need to deny his identification with her, and the feminine, to prove his masculinity.

"Hypermasculinity", the obsession with being a "tough guy", highlights the fact that the roots of male violence lie in rigid and unbalanced sex roles. If our ideas of what is acceptably feminine and masculine were less rigid, boys

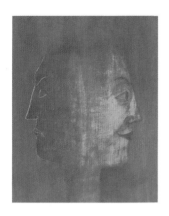

The contemporary Iron John
As exemplified in the Grimm
brothers' character Iron John,
men today need to be in touch
with both the positive and
negative aspects of their
masculinity.

raised by mothers would not have to act in a hypermasculine manner in order to prove they are real men, as it would be acceptable for "real" men to be loving and caring.

Whenever serial killers and psychopaths hit the news headlines, we are told how the mothers of such murderers generally tend to be overbearing, domineering, and hypercritical. Mother is usually blamed for her children's disturbances – witness Norman Bates's mother in Hitchock's classic movie *Psycho* (1960). Yet father is never mentioned. Although a disturbance in the mother-son relationship is a significant factor in the origins of male violence, data suggests that high levels of psychopathic, violent behaviour are frequently linked to a boy having had inadequate – or no – fathering.

Robert Bly uses the Grimm brothers' character Iron John (or Iron Hans in the original), an ancient hairy man, to symbolize what is needed to restore balance to the masculine psychology. Iron John becomes mentor to a young boy, and each event or adventure in Bly's book is seen as a stage in male growth. Iron John is not a savage: he is an "inner warrior", whose task is not one of macho hostility and aggression, but a steady resolve to know and to defend what he loves. Bly believes that a boy's initiation into manhood begins with getting in touch with the "Wild Man" to reconnect himself to Earth: a process that honours the feminine. Bly does not blame mothers for the problems of men. He returns responsibility to fathers and older males for bringing boys into the world of men, and into emotional harmony with women. Through rituals and gatherings – where men provide food and shelter for the boys – a boy can learn that nourishment, tenderness, and nurturing do not come only from a mother, but also from father and other males.

Using myths and legends rather than psychological theory, Bly is saying what many psychotherapists believe: in order to be healthy and whole, a boy has a need for close contact with a reliable, not remote, father – or male role-model – and other men.

Emotions and health

To unblock your ability to love fully, you need to let go of negative emotions such as fear, resentment, hatred, and guilt. Your thoughts, speech, and behaviour are really the only things that can come completely under your control.

Negative feelings of resentment and envy are obstacles that keep many people from achieving harmony within themselves and with others. A positive outlook can, however, be cultivated just as easily as a negative one. Choosing to love can increase your chances of survival under any conditions. This is not simplistically to suggest that by not loving enough you will get seriously ill, but rather that by loving, hatred can be kept from destroying your heart, mind, and life. Your emotions can dramatically affect your body, and your ability to live is not limited by physical health alone.

At the heart of many of the causes of dis-ease lies a person's inability openly to express their pain and outrage, and to have their feelings validated and contained. Evidence suggests that bottling up one's feelings simply forces the emotions to find an outlet of expression somewhere else in the body: stiffness in the joints, pain in the head, neck, or tumours to vital organs. In this sense, our body is acting as an emotional map, charting territory that needs our urgent care and attention.

Traditionally, orthodox (conventional) doctors avoided considering how a person's attitudes can shape their life. While modern medicine has gained much power over certain diseases through drugs and innovative surgery, it has all but forgotten about the potential strength within the patient. As medicine became more technologically advanced, it cast out all non-scientific information that was not easily quantified, and the patient's emotional history grew less and less important.

Our minds do not act only through conscious choices, as in how well we eat, exercise, and take care of ourselves. Our emotions can also directly affect our body tissues, without any awareness on our part. We do not yet fully understand all the ways in which brain chemicals are related to the emotions, but what is clear is that our state of mind has an immediate and direct influence on our physical state of health. Consider some everyday expressions such as, "He's a pain in the neck", or, "You are breaking my heart". Our body responds to the mind's conscious and unconscious messages.

Many enlightened physicians believe that "passive" emotions such as grief, feelings of failure and helplessness, and suppression of anger can cause the production and over-secretion of certain hormones. These hormones can suppress the immune system, which may then lead to diseases such as cancer. Therefore, before we can change what happens to our body we first need to address and understand our emotions.

The way we react to stress and cope with life's problems appears to be more critical than the stress or the problem itself. The feeling of helplessness when associated with stress is a most common cause of disease. Consider the woman who feels trapped in the misery of an unhappy relationship or unfulfilled life, and who has to internalize her stress. Compare this with the kind of stress induced by choosing tasks such as competitive sports or a rewarding career, which is considered normal and healthy. Stresses we choose (such as rock-climbing, or other difficult challenges), evoke a totally different response from stresses we would like to avoid but cannot.

Stress is partly determined by the society in which we live, partly by our own temperament. Cultures and people that have high expectations, material or otherwise, are more likely to experience life as stressful. There may even be a link with cancer, though it is as yet unproven.

If you can give vent to your feelings, you are more likely to stay in good health. Not expressing emotional needs when they first appear can set in train an imbalance in the body, rendering it vulnerable to ill health.

The complexities and causes of serious dis-eases do not all originate in the emotions. Other factors such as genes

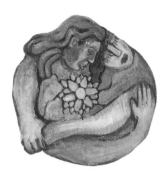

A good hug
Whether for comfort or congratulation, a hug can say more than a thousand words. Emotional outlets, when we show our feelings, without being embarrassed or threatened, help to keep destructive emotions at bay and relieve stress.

and cancer-producing agents (carcinogens) are important. But this does not explain why many people who are genetically prone to cancer, or have been heavily exposed to carcinogens, still do not develop the disease. We need to understand and learn more about the connection between emotions and body in order to prevent the seeds of dis-ease from growing.

An inner stillness and peace of mind, which may be achieved through loving relationships, the practice of yoga, meditation, and therapy, can help to create a healing environment in our bodies. The first step is to understand how our emotions are linked to our body's potential for disease. An understanding of this connection can empower us to change, and to achieve inner peace with ourselves and with others.

WOUNDED EMOTIONS OF WOMEN AND MEN

Women often complain that men do not understand why they feel so upset. And men, confounded by women's reactions, carry on wondering why. Marion Woodman, writing in *The Ravaged Bridegroom* (1990), told of addressing a conference with Robert Bly (author of *Iron John*) in 1988, where she saw in a flash one of the fundamental problems between the sexes. She asked the audience what they associated with "mother". The women instantly responded with words such as "nurturing, cherishing, enfolding, giving, caring". Not a man spoke. Finally, when they were urged to, they roared, "devouring, demanding, manipulative, suffocating, castrating". The women's one-sided and unbalanced attitude had aroused the negative mother in the men, and that apparently simple word "mother" had polarized the sexes.

The dark, shadow side of men is well-documented. Their exploitation of the Earth's resources, their obsession with war, and the devaluation and humiliation of women and the feminine, are undeniable. It is in the world of power, relationships, and sexuality that the differences between women and men seem their most polarized and graphic. Rape and violence against women is reportedly on

Stress scape
Responses to stress differ, depending on the choices we are able to make. The challenge of the "stress" we choose, such as a hard walk on a blustery day, can be exhilarating and uplifting. Whereas stress we wish to avoid, but cannot, may lead to depression and illness.

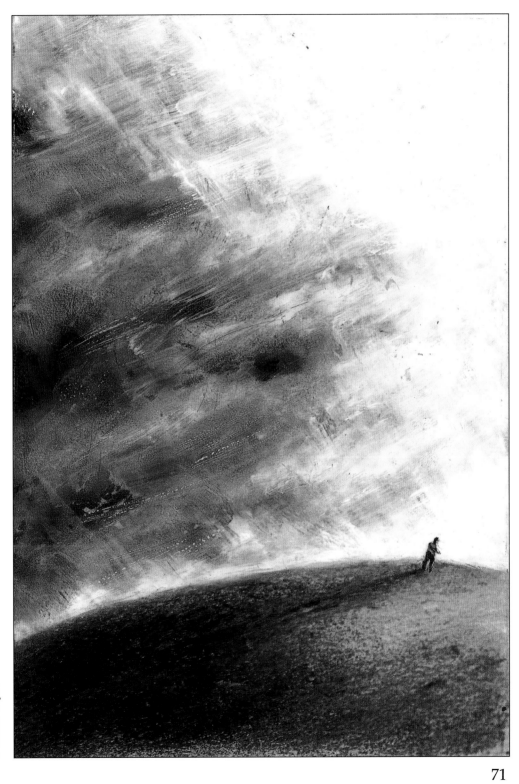

Danielle Blyde

the increase; a backlash appears in the guise of movies and novels such as *Thelma and Louise* (1991) and *Dirty Weekend* (1992), by Helen Zahavi, where the heroines assert themselves in particularly violent ways. Misogyny – the hatred of women – remains deeply ingrained in the psyche of Western culture; the most popular movies tend to be those whose themes either portray women as being poisonous and dangerous, notably *Fatal Attraction* (1987) and *Basic Instinct* (1992), or "slasher" movies, where the victims of horrible crimes are always female. Two recent books, *Backlash* by Susan Faludi (1992) and *The Undeclared War Against Women* (1992) by Marilyn French, have attempted to expose society's hidden misogyny, which continues beneath the apparent liberation women now enjoy and the gains they have made.

How we are raised and emotionally conditioned can contribute to misogyny and violence against women. Early emotional development involves the embodying of the psychologies of our first caregivers. To change the psychology of individuals we need to move toward balance between the feminine and masculine in early care. We must heal the psychological split between women and men. And this needs to begin from birth.

STEPS TO HEAL THE PSYCHOLOGICAL IMBALANCE THAT LEADS TO DISHARMONY BETWEEN WOMEN AND MEN:

• Equal involvement of both parents – vital in the raising of children – or, in the absence of the father, a consistent male role-model

• Through developing a closer connection with his child, the father's, or male role-model's, psychology will alter through his inevitable feelings of vulnerability and anxiety, which are all part of opening up and learning about nurturing

• A son will embody his father's, or role-model's qualities, see them as necessary in his world, too, and bring them to his future intimate sexual relationships and family life

• Two parents – female and male/yin and yang –
representing the power to please or withhold, will
balance and modify the all-powerful, castrating
image of mothers

Imagine the wealth of possibilities! Relationships between
women and men that are built not on fear, betrayal, or solidarity in opposition to the other, but on love, sharing,
harmony, and intimacy. A celebration of the differences,
leading to more connection and union rather than alienation and separation.

EMOTIONS AND THE BREATH

The breath is a bridge connecting mind and body. It is the
door between the conscious and the unconscious, restoring
our natural – but sometimes lost – condition of wholeness.
Many dis-eases could be avoided were we to develop
awareness of breathing.

For many years the breath and breathing techniques
have been used to alleviate the pain of childbirth. More
recently, innovative centres such as the Bristol Cancer Help
Centre have found that breathing techniques make an
enormous difference to some patients, for whom all other
approaches have failed.

For body and mind to be balanced, your breath has to be
rhythmical and continuous. It might help to imagine
breathing as the rhythm section in a band or rock group. If
the rhythm keeps changing without reason, then the music
will be out of synch, and sound disharmonious. The same
with breathing. If you hold your breath and breathe irregularly, the supply of oxygen also becomes irregular. This
lowers your energy and tightens your muscles. When your
breathing becomes out of balance, then it can affect your
abdominal muscles and, in turn, the deep-lying muscles
located in the whole abdominal and pelvic area: the whole
body becomes stiff.

Some city dwellers might be worried that if they breathe
too deeply they will just breathe in more polluted air,
which will make them even more unhealthy. However, by

not breathing fully you only make yourself more tense, stiff, and ultimately unhealthy. When you relax and breathe fully, the body is functioning well, and will be in a better position to process and alchemize the toxins that enter you.

EMOTIONAL ATTITUDES EXPRESSED IN THE BREATH AND BODY

Natural breathing rhythms can become distorted from the moment the first breath is taken. If entry into the world is sudden, with the umbilical cord being cut too soon, a baby's experience becomes disconnected through shock, as there is no continuity from being inside the womb to outside. A baby's first thoughts of the world as hostile and unsafe can set a negative pattern for life.

Breathing can also become disturbed through tensions and frustrations during infancy. If a baby's instinctual biological needs do not meet a satisfactory response, then the baby will become frustrated through continued crying, and may start holding the breath.

As we develop, our emotions continue to influence our breathing. Stress, pain, anxiety, fear of rejection and separation, are common causes of restricted, shallow, or rapid breathing. Holding our breath keeps powerful feelings out of consciousness; stiffening the diaphragm pushes these emotions out of awareness.

AWARENESS OF BREATHING

You can improve your awareness of breathing gradually, with practice and patience. It does not necessarily involve breathing techniques, so much as mindfulness (see pp. 28-30) of your breathing, to help you reconnect with what you already know deep inside.

First, you need to begin to notice how you hold your breath when your mind gets fixed on to certain negative thoughts, such as, "I'm useless", or "I'm no good at anything". By putting your attention on the breath you are letting it flow on, and when you become conscious of your feelings, you can give them space to be. If you try to escape from your thoughts they become unwanted house-guests who will not leave you alone until you satisfy their need for

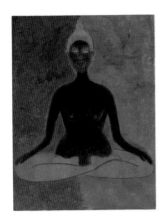

Body puzzle
The lotus is the classic yoga pose for meditation. It demonstrates how the body is perfection itself. The thigh and the sole of the foot fit against each other perfectly.

attention. Instead of trying to suppress your feelings of panic, fear of separation, envy and anger, you can allow them space to be: not to change them, but to relax and feel comfortable with them.

If you breathe rhythmically and regularly, allowing a regular supply of oxygen to enter your blood stream, this will in itself change how you feel, transforming your emotions into feelings of wellbeing.

Slowly this awareness will grow and become part of your experience. Without this awareness, your unconscious thoughts and emotions can make the breath shallow and mechanical.

Through breathing awareness you can identify and heal emotional patterns. You create the body you are living in, and if you are mindful of your breath, body, thoughts, and emotions the easier it will be for you to let go of tension, stiffness, and rigid patterns of thought.

WAYS OF USING THE BREATH TO CONTACT AND RELEASE BLOCKED FEELINGS

Yoga
The practice of yoga is a very powerful way to develop breathing and body awareness. Try not to hold your breath each time a posture, or thought, becomes painful. Once you begin to breathe through the painful sensations, the pain should decrease and your thoughts become still, bringing a sense of relief and openness.

Rebirthing
Another subtle, but powerful, way to connect the breath with your emotions is rebirthing. This method utilizes the breath as a tool to get in touch with and release physiological and psychological stress and unconscious thought patterns from childhood, birth, and earlier.

It is best to learn the technique in the presence of a trained rebirther. You will be asked to lie down and breathe deeply – "conscious connected breathing" –

75

for approximately 45 minutes to one hour to help you release the panic of your first breath. In your breathing you reveal your basic attitudes toward life, and gradually your breath restores itself to the balance and harmony it would have known had it not been for the trauma of your first gasp.

The practice of rebirthing is designed to put you in touch with the pleasure of being alive and allow you to see your birth as an exciting, if frightening, entry into the world. The benefits of rebirthing include easing stressful situations by producing an intuitive sigh of release instead of breath-taking panic. Rebirthing can improve your intimate relationships, partly because they are often controlled by an unconscious fear of separation, caused by the memory of leaving our mother's womb. Through rebirthing you can learn that you are safe in your body, that new beginnings do not mean separation, and that to be alive in your body does not have to mean pain or burden.

AWARENESS OF EMOTIONS AND THOUGHTS DURING BREATHING

• Find a comfortable place to lie down. If the muscles of your body are tense, then your breathing will be shallow, which will make taking a deep breath seem like very hard work
• Lie on your back with your knees bent. Open the space between the shoulder blades by giving yourself a big hug
• Elongate the back of the neck by lifting your head, put your arms by your sides, and hold for a few moments
• Let your whole back release to the floor
• Tune in to your breathing rhythm, without changing it. Just observe your inhalation and exhalation. If it is a long breath say to yourself, "I'm aware it's a long breath", and if it's a short breath say, "I'm aware it's a short breath". You can also say mentally,

"I am breathing in and thinking this thought", and, "I am breathing out and thinking that thought". At the beginning, this helps to train your mind to be present

• After a while, make the exhalation longer. To expand the exhalation, exhale completely counting all the way through the exhalation, and when you reach the end – let's say you count from 1 to 6 – make it last to 7 or 8.

• At the end of the exhalation, let go and wait for the inhalation to come

• At the end of it there is a moment's pause of being empty, and the new breath comes as a surprise. Allow the new air to enter.

• Be aware of thoughts that make you lose your concentration. It is not a matter of needing to forget them but rather to be neither detached from, or attached to, them

• Become aware of one thought, and recognize its presence. Look at your thoughts, bring them out and relax with them

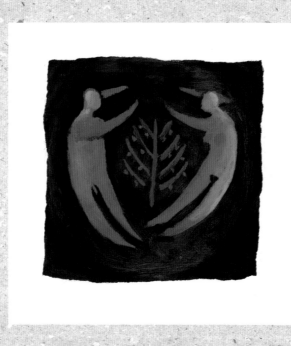

CHAPTER 4

LIFE'S CYCLES
AND RHYTHMS

*"Femininity is defined by the feminine functions,
the fact that we ovulate and menstruate, and we have specific
roles to play in relation to this. If you are
a woman, this is your base feminine rhythm."*
LYNN OSBORNE

Every month the elaborate and beautiful ritual of the menstrual cycle is performed inside millions of women's bodies all over the planet, but taboo, myth, and negativity continue to conceal the positive aspects of this universal experience of menstruation.

Most of the negativity surrounding menstruation arises from a cultural attitude that discounts the bleeding experience and favours the values of childbearing over those of menstruation. Many women are prevented from becoming whole by being regarded as two persons: the good ovulating mother, and the "witch" of menstruation. To speak exclusively of ovulation is psychologically to limit the role of women to this function, and deny that a woman's cycle is a continuum of her past, present, and future. Knowledge about your menstrual cycle and the different energy levels in your body will enhance not only your health and well-being but also your creative abilities, spiritual awareness, intimate relationships, and your whole attitude to your sexuality. Knowing and understanding your feminine rhythms can also help you to maximize and/or minimize the likelihood of conception naturally.

The physiological processes of your cycle

Your cycle can be divided into four phases:

• The menstrual phase (the womb sheds its lining)
• The pre-ovulatory phase (the ovarian follicles ripen and mature)
• The ovulatory phase (the ovary expels a ripe egg)
• Pre-menstrual phase (estrogen and progesterone hormone levels drop)

THE MENSTRUAL PHASE

Menstruation begins a new cycle and marks the end of the previous one. The first day of your bleeding is "Day One". If conception and implantation do not occur between ten and sixteen days after ovulation, your body abandons all its preparations for pregnancy. The whole enriched womb lining collapses and is discharged from the womb amid blood loss. It can take anything from three to seven days for the womb to go through this process. Some women have short, light periods, while others have longer, heavier ones. It is an individual response. As the period ends the womb is ready for the next fertility cycle, and a new opportunity for pregnancy.

Your fertility and basal body temperature (BBT):
The fertility is low straight after the period commences, but this infertile phase is extremely variable in length. If you have a short cycle it may hardly exist at all, because you will go from your period straight into your egg-ripening, fertile phase. If you have average monthly cycles the infertile phase may last about two to three days before the vaginal plug disperses and the fertile mucus starts to appear. If you have long cycles it could be many days before your body ripens another egg.

Inside every woman is an "inner ocean" of cervical and vaginal secretions that change in consistency, quantity, and colour with each of the different phases of the cycle. During the menstrual phase your estrogen levels remain low, which means you may feel dry in the vagina, either with no mucus or with "infertile" mucus, which is scant, sticky, and opaque.

As the result of hormone activity your temperature is low during the less fertile phases. Use a sensitive fertility thermometer (see p. 86) to take your BBT.

THE PRE-OVULATORY PHASE

At some point after your period, the follicle and egg for the new cycle will start ripening and you will become fertile. To start off a new fertility cycle your brain must trigger release of a hormone called follicle-stimulating hormone (FSH), which travels to your ovaries and stimulates one of the many follicles here to ripen and release its egg.

A variety of situations can cause your brain to trigger the release of this hormone erratically, so affecting your fertility hormone pattern, causing irregular periods or sometimes even stopping them. Emotional and physical stress, anxiety, ill health, travelling, excessive dieting and exercise can all affect the patterns. Once the stress is reduced and conflicts are resolved the cycle usually settles down and regulates itself.

Your fertility and basal body temperature (BBT):

Once your egg starts to ripen, the ovaries produce increasing levels of the hormone estrogen, which in turn produces increasing levels of fertile mucus. You may feel increasingly wet around the vagina as your mucus changes to the fertile type. It increases in quantity and becomes thinner and milkier. Your temperature may still remain low.

THE OVULATORY PHASE

There are thousands of follicles in your two ovaries, each containing a primary egg cell, waiting to be stimulated to full maturity. Initially the ovaries respond to FSH by ripening several follicles, but gradually one is selected and primed to become the dominant follicle for that cycle, and the others recede. It takes from five to six days for the chosen follicle to complete its final growth spurt in the ovary, to the point where it bursts to release its egg at ovulation.

Imagine the miracle that follows! An ovary is caressed by a fallopian tube and the sensitive fimbria at the end of the tube are poised over it, ready to suck the egg up when it is released. As a follicle ripens, your ovaries produce more

81

estrogen and prepare your womb for fertility. Estrogen manages repair of the womb lining after menstruation; it opens the cervical opening to admit sperm to the womb, and it causes the cervix to produce fertile mucus, which enhances sperm life. This mucus attracts sperm; it is alkaline, which protects them against vaginal acidity (which normally kills them), and it is also very rich in nutrients that prolong sperm life for several days inside the reproductive tract. At first your mucus appears white and creamy, but by the time the egg is ready for release it is wet, clear, and stretchy, like raw egg white.

To achieve ovulation a new hormone is needed – luteinizing hormone (LH). Its release, too, is triggered by your brain. It surges into the bloodstream for a day, and acts like a needle to prick the taut follicle, causing it to burst and release its egg. The egg is sucked up into the fallopian tubes, to be made available to any waiting sperm. The egg now has a natural life of two days, unfertilized.

The empty follicle then changes to a gland, called the corpus luteum, which produces the next-needed hormone – progesterone. This is the pregnancy hormone, designed to look after the egg in case it is fertilized. Dominating your cycle for the next two weeks, it inhibits all future ovulations, prepares your womb for possible pregnancy by enriching its lining, and raises your body temperature for the two week period. Then it glues up the fertile mucus to form a plug in the cervix, sealing off the womb from infection and further invasion of sperm. If you have intercourse in the fertile mucus phase while the cervix is still open, you may become pregnant.

Your fertility and basal body temperature (BBT):
This is the most fertile time of the cycle, because of the open cervix and the presence of the fertile mucus, which can keep sperm alive for several days inside the cervix. Your mucus begins to become clearer and more watery, and at the estrogen peak, just before ovulation, it is slick and glossy and you may be able to stretch an unbroken, shimmering thread of it between your thumb and forefinger.

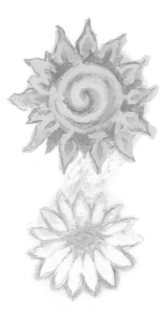

Working with Nature

Conscious conception does not mean controlled conception, it is working with – not against – the laws of Nature, and it is an acceptance of what is and letting be, rather than manipulative fertility.

This kind of mucus is called "Spinnbarkeit" (or "Spinn"). The last day of wet, clear mucus is called Peak Day – the peak of fertility. After ovulation is complete, estrogen levels gradually lessen and the fertile mucus dries up, making pregnancy unlikely.

Once ovulation occurs, progesterone is released and this raises your body temperature. A sensitive fertility thermometer will register the reading (see p. 86).

PRE-MENSTRUAL PHASE

This is the time just before your next period when you may feel depressed, tense, bloated, and uncomfortable. You may experience aches and pains in your back or breasts for several days before you begin to bleed.

Your fertility and basal body temperature (BBT):
Your temperature is low, you will be dry around your vagina, and conception is unlikely.

YOUR CYCLE DURING AND AFTER PREGNANCY

If a sperm penetrates the outer crust of your egg on its journey down the fallopian tube, then fertilization takes place and a new life is conceived. The new baby's cells start multiplying rapidly as they are propelled toward your womb. This journey takes a few days, and during this time the womb lining becomes thick and soft, with a rich blood supply. By about the eighth day after ovulation and conception, the fertilized egg is usually well attached to the womb lining; implantation has taken place.

Once pregnancy is achieved, the cycle of menstruation is suspended until some time (usually a few months) after the birth. Ovulation and menstruation may be further suspended if you breast-feed. But breast-feeding does not necessarily act as a contraceptive, as is sometimes believed, and ovulation may occur without there being a period, making it possible for you to conceive again. You should use contraception or natural fertility awareness (see pp. 84-93) if you do not wish to conceive again straight away.

Knowing your own menstrual rhythms is a great advantage, even after you have conceived. During pregnancy, ultrasound is frequently used to determine the exact date of conception, and the expected date of birth. However, gestational age based on good menstrual records, supported by a pelvic examination in the first few months of pregnancy, may be more reliable and safer than ultrasound. Most units use ultrasound routinely and it can be helpful to the obstetrician to determine the baby's progress, but until its safety is proven and there is some evidence to suggest that it is not necessarily harmless, it should only be used when there is a real medical need, and not for determining the due date. In any case the estimate of 40 weeks gestation is only an average time and a healthy pregnancy may vary in length from 36-44 weeks, although very few obstetricians will allow a pregnancy to run over 42 weeks without some intervention.

During pregnancy there is a definite cyclical relationship going on between the mother and the baby: the mother begins to tune in to the baby's cycle, allowing the pregnancy to happen without "doing" anything, and the baby also tunes in to the cycle of the mother's body; her heart beat, her rhythms, and how she moves and breathes.

Conscious conception and contraception

"Conscious conception", a term coined by Jeannine Parvati Baker and Frederick Baker, is about going with the flow of life – being willing to be pregnant if you become pregnant – rather than a foolproof method of preventing conception.

Fertility awareness is the quintessential holistic approach to one's sexuality, since it requires developing a greater awareness of one's desires on a physical, mental, emotional, and spiritual level. The emphasis is on being conscious of your own body and fertility in the present moment, and any practice that nourishes awareness of staying with the present will enhance your self-development. Knowing your feminine rhythms can do more than connect you to the Earth's seasons and improve your health; it also helps you maximize and or minimize the likelihood of conception. The term "conscious conception" was coined in the belief that the term "birth control" is misleading. It implies that we can exercise authority over people and Nature, a concept that originated around the time of the Industrial Revolution. The body is not the same as a machine, and we cannot "control" anything to do with life: we can only manipulate and sometimes destroy it. A woman's fertility happens whether or not we pay attention to it, so the way to work is with – not against – the laws of Nature.

Through fertility awareness you can increase the elements of communication, honesty, and sharing in your sexual relationship with your partner, as it offers the space for you as a couple to communicate in deeper ways. If you can talk to your partner about such things as vaginal mucus, you can talk to him about practically everything!

Largely because of the Pill, natural methods of contraception have become eclipsed. Conscious conception (natural) methods are healthier; they however take more careful planning, more motivation, and may not be 100% effective. Just as you know when you are hungry, thirsty, or tired, with practice you can also learn accurately to sense when you are fertile. As a woman you need to become familiar with the subtle messages transmitted daily via your mind-body-spirit through your vaginal mucus, cervix, body temperature, and your feelings, moods, sexual desires, and dreams.

HOW TO PRACTICE CONSCIOUS CONCEPTION

Vaginal mucus

Vaginal mucus is an ever-changing secretion of the cervix. It may be helpful to think of it as your "internal ocean". The cervix secretes two types of mucus: fertile and infertile. Fertile mucus is slippery, clear, translucent, stretchy, similar to raw egg white, sometimes tinged with pink, yellow, brown or red, sweet to the taste, sweet to the smell, and it creates a distinct feeling of wetness. Infertile mucus is scant, sticky, and opaque, causing a feeling of "dryness" in the vagina. The components of the mucus change according to your hormones, so that at times in your cycle there will be more fertile- than infertile-type mucus, and at other times vice versa.

To become aware of your mucus you will need to become accustomed to its touch, taste, smell, and feel; all part of getting to know your own body and becoming comfortable with yourself. The best way to examine your mucus is to squat or lie comfortably, breathe consciously, with your vagina as relaxed as your mouth (if your mouth is relaxed then your vagina will be too). Insert one or two fingers into your vagina and gently pull down a sample of your inner fluids. It is unnecessary to do this if mucus has already appeared on your underwear. Suffering from a cold, vaginal infections, or experiencing sexual arousal, will increase the amount of mucus and alter its consistency.

Your cervix

You can also use this time to determine the status of your cervix. With your fingers gently inside your vagina, reach and touch the tip of your cervix. Your cervix feels as firm as your lips when you are fertile, and as firm as the tip of your nose when you are not.

Body temperature

Your basal body temperature (BBT) is the temperature your body drops to when you are sleeping, and hormonal changes cause this base temperature to rise and fall. To record these subtle changes, you will need a sensitive fertility, or basal body thermometer (available from most chemists or drug stores and fertility awareness teachers).

Your temperature will be lower from the beginning of your period until ovulation. Rising progesterone causes your temperature to rise an average of .6 degrees Fahrenheit over your pre-ovulatory phase temperature.

For greater accuracy, when you are using your temperature as an indication of ovulation, take the reading at the same time as examining your mucus. You must record three consecutive temperatures that are .6 degrees higher than your temperatures prior to the rise. After you have recorded the rise on the morning of the third day, you know that you have ovulated. This coincides with your

Natural cycles
The emotional and physical changes that form part of every woman's life can be compared to the cycles of Nature. Each of these changes, like the seasons, has its own beauty, positive and negative qualities, strengths and weaknesses.

86

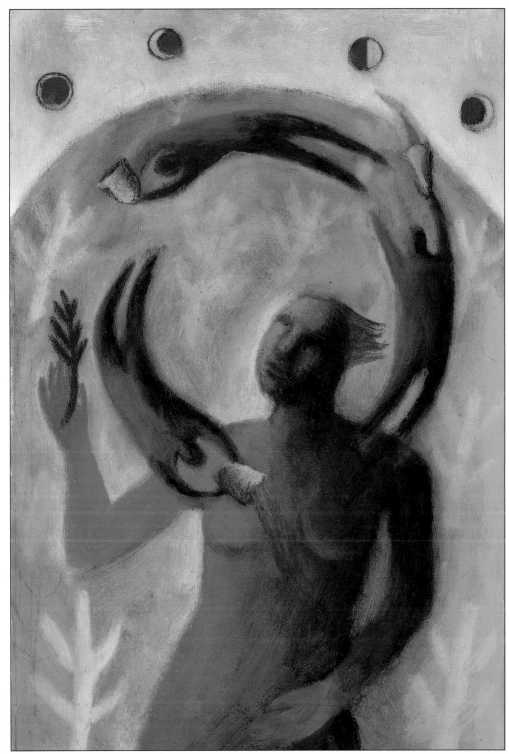

Giovanna Pierce

mucus drying up and your cervical opening hardening, lowering, and closing.

Feelings, moods, sexual desire, and dreams

There are distinct changes in a woman's emotions during the corresponding poles of ovulation and menstruation, and through awareness of your cycle you will gradually become familiar with the rhythms and patterns of your inner and outer life. An understanding of this will help you to nurture your own needs, and respond appropriately to the needs of others.

POINTS TO REMEMBER

If you are relying solely on fertility awareness for your contraception, you and your partner should consult a natural fertility awareness teacher, who can offer support, professional advice, and ensure that you both understand the natural fertility method fully. In addition, you and your partner should be aware of the following:

• Emotional and physical stress, an inadequate diet, and ill health, can disrupt your cycle, making it difficult to "read"

• It is easier to determine when ovulation has occurred than it is to know when it will happen, as your temperature rises noticeably after ovulation

• Ovulation can happen at any time from 12 to 16 days before menstruation. Most women ovulate about two weeks before their next period, not 14 days after the previous one

• Preparation for your next ovulation happens before the menstruation that introduces your new cycle, which explains why, occasionally, women become pregnant from intercourse at menstruation

• Your cycle can change its own rules and confound scientists and doctors, who usually hold the view that the "normal" cycle is 28 days long. Ovulation can happen at almost any time of the cycle under a stimulus such as the presence of a desired love,

artificial lighting, or the strong wish for a child
• Most of us do not have 28-day cycles, and ovulation, with or without a detectable temperature rise, can occur at any time in the cycle, or even twice in the same cycle

Conventional methods of contraception

In an ideal world all available contraception would be 100% effective, 100% safe, and 100% natural. As this is not the case, each and every woman will have to make continual decisions, weighing up the pros and cons of each method and how appropriate it is for her particular situation. As much as we all strive to be healthy and would prefer to practice an holistic method of birth control, this has to be weighed against the possible trauma of conceiving an unwanted child. While it is physically more healthy to practice conscious conception, an abortion would negate any positive benefits. You should discuss your concerns and the options open to you with a family planning adviser, gynaecologist, midwife, or holistic health practitioner who has specialist knowledge in fertility. The important thing is that you make your decision from an informed position.

BARRIER METHODS

These are simple to use and unharmful, as well as being effective (97% effective, if used properly and with spermicidal jelly or cream). They are the male condom, the female condom, and the diaphragm (for women).

The use of male and female condoms has escalated recently, since they offer some protection against the transmission of venereal infections, including AIDS. However it must be stressed that there is no foolproof method of contraception that offers 100% protection against the HIV virus and AIDS.

The disadvantages of barrier methods:
• You need to plan ahead or interrupt your lovemaking
• The spermicide is rather messy
• Some men and women find they are allergic to the

latex in condoms and to some spermicides
- They may reduce sensitivity/pleasure
- Condoms have been known to break during intercourse

INVASIVE METHODS

In contrast to barrier contraceptives, there are methods of contraception that – while being more effective – carry a risk to the health of the woman using them.

The intra-uterine contraceptive device (IUCD or coil)

This is a thin piece of bent plastic, metal or some other material, that is inserted into the uterus for months or years, to prevent pregnancy. An IUCD must be fitted by a qualified nurse or doctor and is about 96% effective.

Physicians have yet fully to explain how this device works. It may cause an inflammation of the uterine lining that probably prevents implantation of a fertilized egg.

The main complications of using an IUCD

- If you become pregnant with an IUCD in place there is a 50% chance of miscarriage. Therefore, if a pregnancy happens a woman should have her coil removed immediately to prevent infection.
- There is increased risk of an ectopic pregnancy (when a fertilized egg implants itself in the fallopian tube instead of the womb). This can mean the loss of the affected fallopian tube.
- Women with multiple partners, who use IUCDs have a higher incidence of pelvic infection, leading to Pelvic Inflammatory Disease (see pp. 187-8).

If you have abdominal pain or tenderness, fever, or unusual discharge, seek the early advice of your doctor. If you have never had a child – and want to – you should not consider using an IUCD, because of the greatly increased risk of pelvic infection that can lead to sterility. (At present hundreds of women in the US and the UK are seeking legal compensation against the manufacturers of the Dalkon Shield.) Many childless women – allegedly made sterile from its use – say that had they been told the risks before-

90

hand they would never have chosen to use the coil as a method of birth control.

Despite these risks, about 50 million women throughout the world use the IUCD with no complications; however, it is worth stating the facts to help you make a well informed decision.

Hormonal contraceptives

The Pill, available since 1961, was part of the sixties revolution in the liberation of youth culture. The Pill offers nearly 100% protection against pregnancy, but, like many innovations which at first seemed to offer so much freedom, it has been at a cost to the health of a great many women.

The most common contraceptive pills combine synthetic forms of the hormones estrogen and progesterone, and are taken daily on a monthly cycle. The estrogen released by the pill raises the woman's estrogen levels to simulate pregnancy, which means that while she takes the pill her ovaries are relatively inactive and no egg is released. The progesterone increases the viscosity of cervical mucus and alters the development of the uterine lining.

The effects of the Pill are said to be reversible: if you want to become pregnant you simply stop taking it. However, in reality many women find it takes several cycles before they become regular again. The long-term incidence of infertility is higher for women who have taken the Pill, particularly for those who have not had any children. The problem is that it is difficult to assess the risks and side-effects since much of the information appears contradictory. One thing is for sure, many women experience nausea, headaches, weight gain, and loss of libido. They may also be prone to increased risk of blood clots, high blood pressure, cervical cancer, thrush, depression, venereal infections, gall bladder disease, epilepsy, and liver tumours. There is also evidence that the Pill generally undermines the immune system, since women on the Pill suffer from more viral infections than others.

THE MENOPAUSE AND CONTRACEPTION

Menopause (see pp. 114-17) is the tapering off of a woman's fertility wherein ovulation, and therefore periods, occur infrequently and further apart until they stop altogether. It is very common to skip three or four periods, and then ovulate and get a period two weeks later. Although fertility does decline when a woman reaches her forties, it is still possible for her to conceive. Even if you have periods irregularly it is still a good idea to chart your temperature and cervical mucus, which can warn you of ovulation when it does come. It is only considered safe for a woman in her menopause to stop using precautions when she has not had a period for two years.

As the risks of pregnancy decline, you may wish to opt for the diaphragm, condom, or natural fertility methods rather than the Pill. Since the menopause produces its own hormonal fluctuations it would be unwise to upset this further by introducing synthetic hormones into a menopausal woman's bloodstream.

HOW TO RECONCILE ORTHODOX AND NATURAL METHODS OF CONTRACEPTION

Like everything else in life we should aim to bring a balance in evaluating even the most difficult of decisions. The following are suggestions as to how you might combine the use of orthodox and natural methods of birth control:

• If you do not have a regular sexual partner, are breastfeeding, or in the menopause, it may be more appropriate to use a barrier method rather than take the Pill. If you are using the Pill, diaphragm, or IUCD but do not have a regular partner you should always use a barrier method, such as the female or male condom as well, for some protection against the HIV virus, AIDS, and other sexually transmitted diseases. Note, however, that there is no foolproof method of contraception that also gives 100% protection against the HIV virus and other sexually transmitted diseases

• When using barrier methods, use this time – without running the risk of becoming pregnant – to become more aware of your fertility cycle

• If you are taking the Pill, ensure that your health remains in optimum condition to compensate for the effects that it might have. Have regular health checks at a Family Planning/Well Woman clinic. and consult an alternative health practitioner (such as a homeopath or acupuncturist) to help boost your health at all levels. Eat a highly nutritious diet (there are also vitamins and supplements available specifically for women taking the Pill), stop smoking, and cut down on alcohol

• If you wish to become pregnant it is advisable to come off the Pill for at least 6 months before conceiving. During this time use barrier methods, and become aware of your natural cycle. You can eventually use this knowledge to enhance the time you wish to conceive. It may also be helpful to consult a pre-conceptual counsellor

• If you are using an IUCD try to become more aware of any changes in your body, such as a high fever, and particularly any pain or sensitivity in the abdominal area. Maintain a high level of health so that in the event of any infection you will be in much better condition to fight it. Regular consultations with a homeopath, acupuncturist, or traditional Chinese doctor will help to boost your general level of health

• If you have never been pregnant, but wish to be at some later stage of your life, when choosing your contraceptive method always consider how it may affect your future fertility

"Women's bodily functions are pathologized because they 'interfere' with masculine things. If you have to take time off work, then periods are seen as negative. We need to give permission to women to be different during this time, but on an unconscious level. It is allowing rather than doing. Denial of the process is masculine."
BENIG MAUGER, ANALYTICAL PSYCHOTHERAPIST

Menstrual truths

The masculine principle in medicine sees women essentially as breeders with an ovulatory function, so their other half – the menstrual side – is neglected. This neglected bleeding has been turned into a sickness, which doctors call pre-menstrual syndrome – PMS.

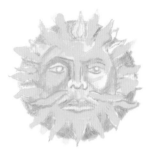

The negativity and fear surrounding menstruation is reflected in slang words such as "the curse" and "on the rag". The onset of your period may be an inconvenience, particularly if you are travelling or undertaking some form of sport. You may feel irritable and extremely sensitive just before your period begins, and experience menstrual cramps (which may vary at different stages of life). Cramps may range from mild and hardly noticeable to very strong spasms in the abdomen and pelvis, the inner thighs, and the lower back. Sometimes they are so intense that they can induce nausea and vomiting.

Sun and Moon
Robert Bly, poet, author, and storyteller, points out how divisive it is when we make such claims as; "The Earth is female", and "God is male", because he believes that these statements reinforce the split that already exists between the feminine and masculine. It is traditionally accepted that feminine cycles are linked with the moon and many believe men to be more aligned to the sun. Perhaps even symbolism has become too gender-rigid.

You may feel that your body has become bloated (due to hormonal changes and water retention), and that you have become clumsy, "spaced out", and forgetful. You may also get urges to eat sweet, "comfort" foods.

Emotionally you may experience a wide range of moods just before your period, varying from depression and sadness to irritability and sensitivity. When you cannot express, or are out of touch with, these feelings you may be diagnosed as suffering from pre-menstrual syndrome (PMS). But it is quite natural to experience a surge of wide-ranging emotions at this time.

There are few accounts of what women normally, or positively, experience during the cycle. More often the negative effects of these profound rhythmic changes are described, alongside the statistics to prove them (see box p. 96).

THE DENIAL OF MENSTRUATION SYMBOLIZES THE DEMISE OF THE FEMININE

The feminine rhythms and healing powers of the menstrual cycle are fundamental to harmony, balance, and wellbeing: their denial reflects and symbolizes the rejection of feminine and spiritual values in all aspects of modern life.

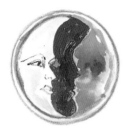

The taboo surrounding menstruation has been one of the most successful and powerful means to undermine the self-acceptance and confidence of women. If positive values were assigned to menstruation, then menstrual distress might ease. What would happen if pre-menstrual syndrome was referred to as pre-menstrual strength? Some PMS is however pathological in its extreme expression, and a variety of therapeutic approaches (including psychotherapy) are appropriate.

Knowledge of what happens to a woman during labour – combined with breathing awareness, a sensitive environment, and freedom to move around during contractions – has helped to revolutionize the birth experience for both women and babies. Women determine their own labour experience, but techno-obstetrical backing is still available. A change of attitude to menstruation and the menopause would bring about similar positive benefits, and it is at least worth a try to see what a change of attitude would uncover.

New approaches are already being applied to the forgotten feminine experience of menstruation. Just as there are natural birthing classes everywhere, workshops are beginning to appear that explore "creative menstruation". The Menstrual Foundation in California, and Hygieia College in Utah offer workshops, products, and publications enhancing the positive and creative aspects of menstruation and menopause. It is hoped that similar centres will be established worldwide.

THE MOMENT OF TRUTH

Most women who are admitted to mental hospital for emotional crises, who commit suicide, or who carry out violent offences, do so during the paramenstrum – the four days before the period and the four days after. Perhaps this period is a "moment of truth" in a woman's life, the significance of which is denied and continually repressed month after month. Let's say you are a woman who is unhappy with her life, who has blocked out past trauma and abuse, but who now wants a more peaceful existence.

You suppress your feelings about your past, your life, your partner, your family, and the pressures on you to conform to society's expectations. Then – at the moment of truth in the paramenstrum – all your forgotten and repressed feelings emerge and rise to the surface, particularly repressed feelings of need. In our society you as a woman generally are expected to take care of other peoples' needs, and this time of the month can be particularly difficult if your own needs have not received enough attention. Because such emotions are given no other language, you cannot express them outwardly, so they hurt you inwardly – expressing themselves either in body-language, illness, or accident-proneness.

During menstruation you have less ability to suppress your true inner desires, vulnerabilities, and your power, which you may do at other times of the month. The time of your bleeding may be the moment of truth and self-healing, which – if consistently suppressed – can become the moment of rage and despair.

TUNING IN TO YOUR FEMININE RHYTHMS

Your cycle (see pp. 80-3) has two poles of culmination – ovulation and menstruation – and through awareness of your emotions, the passage of change from one pole to the other will become easier. There are many possibilities of experience if you open yourself to your feminine rhythm. If you become aware of the different emotions surrounding your cycle, you will be able to perceive rhythms deeply rooted in your bodily experience. Failure to perceive these rhythms may isolate you from processes that can bring balance, self-healing, and harmony. Even if you do not enjoy your cycle, it will certainly help if you become more aware of the different feelings you experience. Periods are a sign of a healthy body in tune with Nature.

If you detach yourself from your feelings and regard menstruation as an inconvenience or illness, then your detachment ensures that the changes in your cycle remain merely bodily ones, which may force them to express themselves in the body-language of illness symptoms. Being in

PMS – the facts and figures
- *PMS is the commonest condition for which American women consult doctors*
- *84% of crimes of violence committed by women were during the "premenstrum" (the days just before the period)*
- *In school examinations taken during the paramenstrum (the four days before the period and the four days after) girls' academic performances can suffer*
- *In one study 45% of 276 female acute psychiatric patients were admitted to hospital during the paramenstrum*
- *Sickness among women in industry is greatest during menstruation*
- *Women are more accident-prone during the paramenstrum*

tune and flowing with the rhythms of your cycle can lead to a new and enlightened sense of independence, which will help you to understand your true self, rather than repress your femininity.

When you begin to look for the positive, and allow and understand the negative aspects of the cycle, you will make some remarkable discoveries:

INCREASED MENTAL AND CREATIVE POWERS

Many women find that just before menstruation their emotions undergo a marked change. If you are not able to welcome the bleeding, you may experience these changes in your personality negatively, as in PMS or depression.

It is a common reaction to think of the period as a nuisance, since many women are prone to the inconvenience and the discomfort of cramps, tender breasts, and feeling bloated. However, experiencing this phase as a "curse", with oversensitivity, pain, and irritability, may also be because you are unaware of your body's deep and instinctual longing for a child. If you can acknowledge and accept such emotions, then the menstrual phase can become a time of developing fertile insights and new relationships. With understanding and awareness of your emotions, a different set of energies can become available to you during menstruation: those of receiving, accepting, and building the potential within you.

As you begin to feel positive about your bleeding, so you will begin to experience unmistakable and powerful changes in your attitude. During bleeding a woman becomes more conscious of her body; she may become more introspective and aware of the fact that another month has passed. Bleeding is a time for reflection and thoughtfulness. The emphasis on regeneration produces an intensity of thought, emotions, and feelings – of all the senses in general. You may find that your senses heighten, including increased awareness of colours, sounds, tastes, and other sensations. You may feel more creative than usual, new ideas may form and you may be able to make work decisions more easily. Positive thought also helps acceptance and love for your body and its functions, which increases your confidence and self-worth. Sadly, many women have negative body images, partly as a result of the constant media barrage of "perfect" models and actresses.

In the past, women healers used their menstrual time as a source of inspiration, when their visions and prophecies became clearer. Psychoanalyst Natalie Shainess has stated that menstruation is the best time for counselling, as it is an optimum time for growth. Whilst bleeding you have an opportunity to get in touch with a deeper, more fundamental layer of your emotional life. Symptoms of physical or emotional disturbance may indicate that there is a conflict between your conscious attitude, and the demands of your true desires and nature. If you can recognize any menstrual distress as an indication of your need to be by yourself, and withdraw psychologically from the demands of your external life, you may be able to re-establish contact with the deeper part of your nature. Many women find it extremely healing to withdraw into themselves, and devote attention to these other sides of their personality.

If a woman has fully acknowledged the meaning of menstruation she is more likely to feel positive, receptive, and accepting around the time of ovulation, since this is the part of the cycle that is most valued in society. Your body is fertile at this time of the month, so you may feel an emotional expansiveness, an abundance of sexual energy, and a new potency in your creative ideas and insights.

As yet, however, the majority of women do not experience ovulation like this, since suppression of the feelings around menstruation leads to suppression of the feelings around ovulation too. When a woman acknowledges all that menstruation brings to the surface only then will she experience the positive aspects of ovulation fully.

SPIRITUALITY AND MENSTRUATION

The spiritual aspect of our cycle is in its symbol of wholeness. Like the cycles of the moon and plants, menstruation represents the regeneration of life. It is a reminder of a woman's rebirth every month, which can make her feel in

Laws of Family Purity
Menstruation is a focal point of an Orthodox Jewish woman's marital relations. During the time of her bleeding and for seven days afterward, the Laws of Family Purity forbid her to have physical contact with her husband. The "ritual impurity" is a spiritual concept, and is restored at the end of her period when she ritually immerses in holy waters, known as the "mikvah". The Laws were designed to be in harmony with a woman's physical, emotional, sexual, and spiritual makeup. The act of separation offers the woman privacy and a time for inward reflection and it protects her gynaecological health. During menstruation, a couple demonstrate their love for each other through non-physical ways. The separation encourages them to develop a friendship, which will find physical expression once the bleeding is over.

The Muslims have similar laws of separation, and the Hindus practice a tradition of separation at menstruation, but it is not a law.

Strange as it may seem, the Laws of Family Purity do not contradict a woman's right to act on her desires during menstruation. What they simply do is to uphold the fact that whether to act on sexual desires or not should be a woman's choice. For many women today – like the women in ancient times – menstruation is a time when they do not wish to be sexual. However, some women still feel unsure of trusting their instincts, therefore the Laws can serve to validate their wish for separation. Similarily, recognizing that the taboo against intercouse during mensturation is founded on superstition not fact can serve to validate those women who wish to make love during their period.

tune with the regenerative processes of Nature.

In the religious teachings of Orthodox Judaism, the Laws of Family Purity (see box left) focus on menstruation as an opportunity for spiritual self-development and deepening the relationship with a partner. Whatever our faith, these Laws have something to teach us. They can help us understand how to use menstruation to deepen our spiritual awareness.

DEEPER INTIMACY WITH YOUR LOVER

Evidence suggests that an increase in sexual awareness and surge of sensuous feelings may be associated with the paramenstrum, although this is not always acknowledged. Masculine science continues to pronounce that it cannot occur, since the human race cannot, or can only rarely, be increased by sex at this "infertile" time.

A woman's increased desire to be intimate with her partner during the paramenstrum might be interpreted as sexual desire, but may actually indicate a wish to relate at a deeper, transcending level with him, and not necessarily the desire for increased sexual intercourse. An increase in sexual awareness implies wholeness and a desire for deeper intimacy, not just heightened lust. There is a type of sexuality of an initiating kind that reaches a peak during the paramenstrum, when our passion and creativity can be aroused in the wider sense of the word.

It is to your advantage – and your partner's – to know when your most sexually sensitive and receptive times are. If your sexual desire increases just before or during menstruation, outside of religious Laws, you should not be inhibited by custom or taboo against lovemaking at this time. Some taboos have undoubtedly arisen from myths, superstition, and some men's fear of women's sexuality. On the other hand, menstruation may be the time you feel least sexually drawn to your partner. If so, use this time to enhance, strengthen, and totally transform your relationship with your partner, by communicating on a deeper, non-physical, level. The choice should be yours, based on what feels right for you, your body, and your health. It is vital for women to be aware of when they themselves feel erotic. For the woman whose religion forbids sexual intimacy during menstruation, it is her choice to abstain, based on her faith.

THE MOON AND MENSTRUATION

The name "menstrual cycle" comes from the Latin "mensis" meaning "month", which also means "moon". Many people believe in a connection between human fertility and the moon, since it seems more than just a coincidence that the average length of a menstrual cycle, 28 days, matches that of the lunar phases.

In ancient Greece, women's periods were said to correspond with the moon's phases. Perhaps, like women in ancient times, we can open ourselves to this lost "lunar rhythm". Women's lunar rhythm was rediscovered by an American worker Edmond Dewan, he advised a woman with a history of irregular cycles to sleep with the light on during the days ovulation was expected. This unconventional course of treatment promoted more regular ovulation by imitating the moon's light and patterns.

The idea was further developed by Louise Lacy in her ground-breaking book *Lunaception* (1976), where she proposed that women have evolved a physiological response to the light and dark cycles of the moon. Lacy kept a daily record of her temperature, behaviour, and general outlook, and observed her vaginal secretions. To duplicate the pre-electric environment of our foremothers Lacy slept in total darkness, except during the middle of her menstrual cycle, when she would sleep with a dim light shining on her.

Gradually, she began to detect a pattern. As she began to harmonize with her body, she could predict accurately peaks and lows of mood, self image, creativity, physical activity, and sexual desire. Lacy's cycle regularized and menstruation became shorter. The connection between the use of the light mid-month, and temperature and mucus increases recorded on her chart, made fertility entirely predictable. By simply observing, Lacy found it was possible to make pregnancy optional. She introduced these practices

"Since my husband has learned to wait for the infertile period of my cycle, he has also learned to wait for me during sexual intercourse, and this has completely transformed our union."
MARY SHIVANANDAN,
NATURAL SEX

"If I could read somewhere that the period is a deeply rewarding and spiritual time, and that other women feel it, then I would allow myself to feel it, too."
ALICE

to other women, who all reported that Lunaception gave them not just a way to make fertility optional but also a sense of spiritual wholeness and wellbeing.

By introducing a rhythm of moon-lit nights, you can help your womb "see" your innate natural rhythm of the lunar cycle. If you increase indirect lighting (moonlight or shaded lamplight) at the time of your anticipated ovulation, not only can you stimulate ovulation but you can also ease menstrual distress. Use this self-knowledge to help enhance your whole life. Knowing your highs and lows can help you to reserve moments of decision to times of physical and mental alertness; you can recognize your times of vulnerability and protect yourself accordingly; you can use the peaks of your moods and creativity to inspire positive interaction between you and your partner.

THE INNATE WISDOM OF THE CYCLE

Through the study of daily and monthly biological body rhythms, doctors have discovered the cyclical patterns of nature. In the past physiologists specializing in body clocks maintained that the best time for a patient to undergo surgery would be the time of day when the surgeon feels at his or her best. However, in 1991 surgeons came to recognize the connection between the outcome of surgery and the monthly ebb and flow of the patient's hormones – especially female patients' hormones. It is in the timing of breast cancer surgery that precise knowledge of where a woman is in her cycle has been found to be most critical. A study carried out by R. Badwe et al. (*The Lancet*, Vol 337, May 25, 1991) at Guy's Hospital in London states that by simply changing the time of breast cancer surgery, 600 lives a year could be saved. Breast tumours grow slowly. They are dependent on estrogen, which builds up in the body from Day Three of the cycle, and stays high until its effect is blocked by progesterone, released on Day Twelve after ovulation (see pp. 80-3). Therefore, the optimum time for surgery is when a woman is either producing low levels of estrogen or high enough levels of progesterone partly to block the action of the estrogen.

"I generally advise women around menstruation to have increased sleep, increased intake of food, especially protein, just prior to and during periods. Also to consciously reduce stress and if possible plan their life so that on the menstruating days there are less demands and activity on the woman and more opportunity to rest."
PAULINE O'DRISCOLL

101

Pre-menopausal women undergoing breast cancer surgery are now advised to schedule their operation for the second half of their menstrual cycle, avoiding Days Three to Twelve. The outcome of an operation is likely to be better after the thirteenth day of the cycle, or on the first two days of the period.

MENSTRUAL DREAMS

In many older civilizations, women slept more than fourteen hours a day during their periods, because a menstruating woman was known to have a special need for rest and seclusion. A similarity between pre-menstrual syndrome and dream-deprivation was first noted in *The Biology of Dreaming* (1967) by Ernest Hartmann. He discovered that the changes of the cycle produce an increased need for dream-sleep, and his cure for PMS was a prescription for more dream-sleep.

Confused and energetic dreaming is common during the days leading to menstruation. Dream imagery associated with the menstrual time often features the sea, water, red objects, powerful male animals, and powerful women – goddesses – who reveal solutions to problems. If you are visited by powerful dreams during your period try to write them down. Use these images for meditation, since if the meditations are directed toward, and not away from your period, menstrual distress can be overcome.

SHARED RHYTHMS OF THE CYCLE

A woman's whole body-mind is a sensitive receptor to outside influences. The body gives off hormonal substances called pheromones, which act as powerful chemical messengers (rather like perfume). Women unconsciously respond to the pheromones given off by other women living in close proximity. Women living together in the family home, in colleges and convents, and working together in offices may find that their cycles synchronize.

MENSTRUAL MYTHS

There have always been myths and legends associated with women and menstruation, and millions of people are attracted to the vampire myth. Dracula movies continue to

Patchwork tells a story

American women (settlers and pioneers) would traditionally make a patchwork "album" quilt as a means of recording family events such as birth, the rites of passage through puberty, marriage and menopause, or as a record of the chores of daily life, such as tending to their small holdings. Some quilts such as "friendship" quilts, given to a minister or friend who was leaving the community, and "wedding" quilts given to the bride to celebrate her marriage, were the joint work of many women, who came together at social quilting parties, or "quilting bees", and talked as they created.

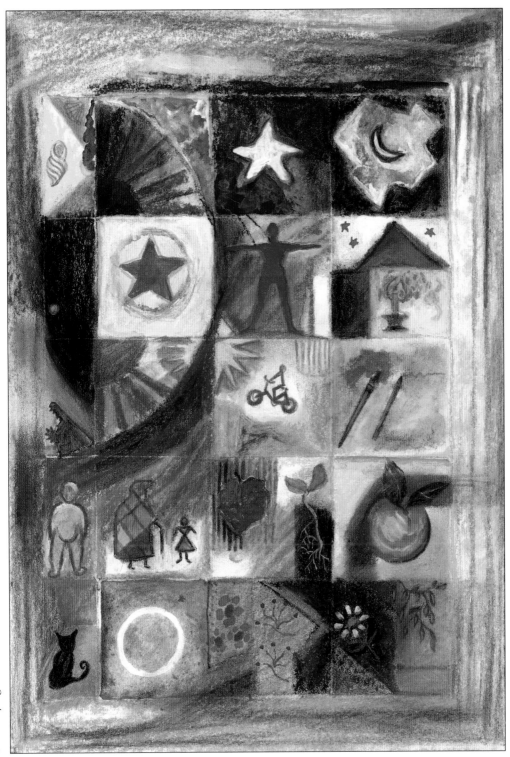

Sara Keeping

be one of the greatest box office successes. Perhaps vampires, with their themes of terror and the shedding of female blood, reflect some of the unconscious conflicts that surround menstruation.

Bram Stoker, the creator of Dracula (1897), was married to a beautiful, but sexually troubled woman, called Florence Balcombe. Perhaps it is safe to assume that as a result of Florence's sexual conflicts she also experienced severe menstrual distress. Is it possible that Florence's conflicts hinted to her husband a formidable force and unacknowledged sexuality, which emanated from her at the time of her bleeding and became the basis of his Dracula idea.

Many of us are familiar with the film image of Dracula wrapped in his cloak with its blood-scarlet lining, going hunting in the full moon for young female victims. Before they are bitten, the women are dull, subservient creatures, but after their blood has been shed, which is always from the neck (as in "neck" or cervix of the womb), they are transformed into independent, and sensuous creatures.

Perhaps, as the vampire myth hints, your periods are not just for the shedding of an unfertilized egg but your bleeding conceals a powerful time of self-healing, creativity, awareness, spirituality, and sexuality, which – when accessed – is designed to enrich and transform the quality of your life.

YOUR PARTNER AND YOUR CYCLE

It is safe to assume that men have cycles, because everything in Nature has a cycle and flows in a cyclical wave or manner. There is a testiculation rhythm in men, that corresponds with the ovulation temperature rise in women. Men's rhythms are waiting to be understood more deeply. A man's inherent rhythm may be difficult to tune in to, since it tends to be overlaid by the menstrual rhythm he picks up from his partner (and in childhood from his mother). If you look for a rhythm in the man who lives with you, you will find it, as there is every indication that your cycles affect him.

104

"If the woman understands her cycle, then she can share it with her partner, which often improves their relationship. The man begins to understand how his partner's changes affect him quite deeply, and begins to understand his own changes in relation to her rhythm. For example, some men experience more erections when their partner is ovulating."
LYNN OSBORNE

The relationship between any man and woman will be inspired to the degree he has comprehended his own fertility cycle and can apply this wisdom to understanding the woman's fertility, imagination, and intuition.

A WORD FOR MEN

You can become in touch with your own cycle simply by tuning in more to your feelings – through massage, dream re-call, meditation, and breathing (see pp. 28-9 and 74-9). You can begin to develop a sensitivity and consciousness to your own rhythm in relation to sperm evolution, testosterone flow, and all of the lost distinctions of the male cycle.

Through observation of your partner's cycle and an understanding of her fertile phases, you will be able to reflect back to her awareness of where she is – at the peak of fertility or in her flow – or somewhere in between on the cycle's continuum (see pp. 80-3). You can encourage your partner to withdraw into her inner sanctum, either by creating an actual space in the home or by encouraging her to create a retreat that is appropriate for her. You understand that her need to withdraw will benefit your relationship, the family, and the community, and you will learn to go inward yourself as you observe her monthly changes.

In educating your son as he enters into sexual maturation as to what it means to support a woman who is in a cycle you will be a role model showing respect for the feminine in your speech and actions.

Menstrual medicine

Menstruation can be seen as a built-in healing mechanism. The original model for healing – turning inward to access the unconscious in order to balance your life – mirrors this natural tendency to turn inward pre-menstrually.

By gaining a greater awareness of fluctuations in our emotions, moods, vaginal fluids, and dreams, we can reclaim the power, without drugs and intervention, to alleviate pre-menstrual syndrome, pre-ovulatory tension, as well as menopausal and other menstrual distress. With you as initiator, intimacy between you and your partner can take on a deeper spiritual dimension, as can the value of forgotten, but innate, "feminine magic" such as intuition, visions, and dreams.

There are several ways you can ease your physical and mental tensions. Yoga, meditation, dream recall, and imaginative thinking are all useful tools to draw upon during the time of your bleeding. Menstrual relaxation (see pp. 107-9) can ease the transition between the various phases of your cycle. It can also help alleviate PMS, improve intimacy between you and your partner, and generally heighten your enjoyment of life.

Guided visualizations are known to help creativity. You can enter relaxation with a problem and find that when you emerge you can see a solution; or you may have a puzzling dream and find that during relaxation you re-dream it, and can relate to it better.

You should not dismiss images of legends and goddesses as useless tales, for they can provide you with a map of self-discovery. They are universal and shared dream images, and a knowledge of them can be the atlas for inner exploration. Increased dream re-call can give your periods meaning, and a feeling of solidarity with women of ancient times. Where the values of sleep, meditation, and relaxation during menstruation have been forgotten, they can now be restored to a woman's life as part of the natural and creative healing processes of her cycle.

With an understanding of menstrual distress come the positive, transformative attributes of increased dreaming, heightened creative energies, and a desire for a deeper, spiritual intimacy with your partner.

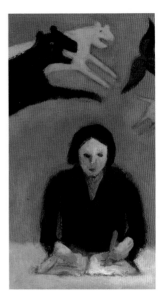

A personal record
One way to celebrate your daughter's menarche is to make her the gift of a special book to be used as her personal journal. Recording thoughts, feelings, and dreams before, during, and after menstruation can help improve awareness of her cycle and ease menstrual tension.

HOW TO RELIEVE MENSTRUAL TENSION

There is inherent wisdom and self-healing that can be gained by understanding the changes in your personality through your cycle. By seeing the patterns that go through your body, and sensing them inwardly, you can release the mental-physical energies called Ovulation, Menstruation, and Inner Man,

106

so that they begin to harmonize with each other. The following suggestions can help you to relieve menstrual tension and to become more in touch with the different phases of your cycle

• With each month that passes, keep a journal of your thoughts and feelings before, during, and after your bleeding times, of both waking events and dreams. You will gradually begin to see the rhythms of your inner and outer life

• During the paramenstrum allow yourself to rest, sleep more, record your dream images, and partake of an extra-nutritious diet. Dreaming, with knowledge of the events of your cycle, can resolve your menstrual and ovulatory distress

• Spend time alone or go for a walk on the days that you bleed, to help provide yourself with space for quiet reflection. Choose beautiful and tranquil settings, preferably near trees, in a park, or by the sea

• If menstruation is a time when sexual contact is uncomfortable or unwelcome for you, use your period as an opportunity to express your love for your partner in non-sexual ways (see also pp. 98-9). This can enhance and deepen your spiritual connection with yourself, and with each other

• Exchange ideas with other women about how you can creatively and imaginatively enjoy and celebrate your bleeding times. This kind of solidarity may be offered by women's groups who specialize in the experience of menstruating

• If demands on your life are so great that you cannot set aside time to spend on yourself, just being aware of yourself at this time of your cycle will help

MENSTRUAL RELAXATION

This relaxation exercise can help to allieviate menstrual tension through an increased awareness of breathing and guided imagery and visualizations. The best time to start menstrual relaxation is during the first quarter of your cycle, when the bleeding has stopped, say on about Day Six or Day Seven. By the time your pre-menstrual feelings come around again you are practised, and day-dreaming or chosen images can take over from the tension. You may find it easier to make a recording of the instructions on a cassette, and play them back while you are going through the exercise. You may wish to do this exercise alone, or possibly a friend or partner can go through it with you.

• Lie comfortably on the floor, your neck slightly propped, and your body covered with a blanket. You may wish to play some relaxing music, or light a candle, or some incense

• Spend a little time getting comfortable and letting go of any muscular tension you become aware of. Close your eyes and let your attention flow between yourself and your breath (see also pp. 28-30)

• Allow your breathing to slow down, perhaps let out a few deep sighs. Feel your spine along the floor, let your shoulders drop, and your jaw and tongue loosen (yawning is great)

• Each time you breathe in, visualize inhaling golden, cleansing light. You are sending healing energy to the whole of your body. Breathe into your abdomen and solar plexus. Let the golden light gradually spread as you breathe out, releasing all the tensions, fears, and worries from the past

• Allow the feeling of warmth and heaviness to spread so that your muscles relax more deeply with every breath

• Send more breath, light, and gentleness to any areas that are feeling tension, discomfort, or pain

• Each time you breath out, allow yourself to relax a little more deeply

• Turn your attention to your feet, wiggling your toes if you need to, really feel the sensation of your feet. Gradually work up your whole body taking in your ankles, shins, calves, slowly, warmly, gently, to your knees and to your thighs and buttocks

- Let warmth and relaxation spread over your belly, the small of your back, the bones of your pelvis
- The whole time remember your breathing. It may even feel as if your breath is breathing you (this will get easier with practice, so do not despair if this does not seem to work at first)
- Continue to let the relaxation and warmth travel over your belly, where the breath is coming and going of its own accord and natural rhythm. Let the relaxation travel to your neck, your jaw, arms, hands, and fingers. Let it travel over your face, which simply rests without expression. Allow the warmth to travel over your eyebrows, brow, and scalp. Try scrunching up your face to release some of the tension
- If thoughts and pictures come into your mind, let them come and let them go. As a thought comes up say to yourself, "I am breathing in, and thinking this thought", and "I am breathing out, and thinking that thought". You can try to visualize white clouds and let your thoughts dissolve into them
- Allow all your tension to drain away to the centre of the Earth, knowing that you are securely and firmly supported

When you are practised at relaxation you can try some simple visualizations at this point.
- Imagine yourself in very beautiful surroundings, very safe, (meadows, the sea-shore, a beautiful room – whatever is right for you). Really let yourself sink and let go in this magic place. Now, visualize your body totally vibrant and healthy
- Stay with your breathing and deep relaxation for as long as you like. You may wish to return quite quickly. But you should take time. Open your eyes very slowly, gradually stretch, and try to keep the relaxation in your body as you get up gently

"I feel that it is terribly important for a woman to start working right from menarche, then she can use her cycle to mature and grow. By the time she has reached her menopause she will know more about who she is."
LYNN OSBORNE

Women's seasons

A rite of passage is one of life's transitions and before we cross a gateway in life, such as puberty or menopause, there may be emotional conflicts that need to be acknowledged, understood, and worked through.

PUBERTY

Puberty is a natural transition from childhood to maturity, and in a young woman it is marked by her first menstrual period, known as "the menarche". In purely physical terms, puberty in a girl is characterized by bone growth, growth of breasts, pubic and underarm hair. Ovulation and menstruation begin near the end of puberty, when a young woman is around twelve, though it can start at any time between the ages of nine and eighteen. It can be a very emotional time, due to the changing hormones and often unconscious anxieties about leaving childhood behind.

Menstruation prepares a woman's body for the possibility of pregnancy every month. If a young woman has already been presented with facts about what will happen, and why, she will cope much better than someone who is totally unprepared. Emerging sexuality should be experienced as a natural stage within the context of her whole life, so that when it happens it can be a gentle transition.

Young women who have positive, accurate information about sexuality are better able to make decisions about sexual matters; they cope better with peer pressure, and thereby feel more able to postpone sexual intercourse for which they do not feel emotionally ready.

As well as being a physical transition, puberty is also a spiritual one. While rites of passage offer an opportunity for transformation, they may also re-evoke repressed trauma or conflict. A young woman may unconsciously greet menstruation in the same way as her mother received hers, and may also make contact with internalized family myths.

INITIATION INTO MENARCHE

The experiences undergone at the menarche are permanently imprinted on the psyche. Many indigenous cultures maintain that menarche is a period of a particular inward

"I dreaded my first period, as it seemed to mark the end of my 'buddy' relationship with my older brother and father. I felt unable to continue to play sports with them after I became a woman, and I sensed my father become distant."
JENNY

Puberty
The creative awakening of puberty is like the "spring" of a woman coming into bloom and fertility.

110

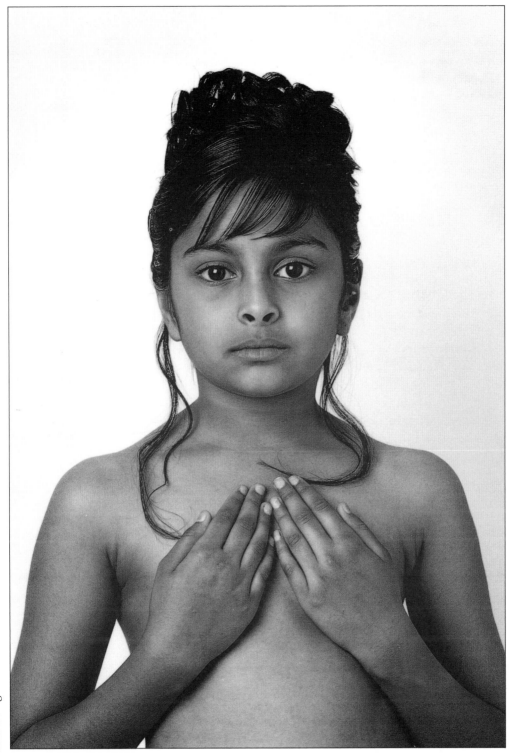

Sian Irving

mental opening, as well as a physical one, during which a young woman may have dreams, and other experiences, that can guide her in later life. The way in which a young woman experiences her menarche may mark the way in which she will experience every period thereafter.

Today Western women would benefit greatly from a ritualization of the menarche, which more primitive societies have met with familial and social rituals. The feminist writer Simone de Beauvoir said how women often feel disappointed if they sense that "nothing has changed" after their first period. Some of the primitive menstrual rites appear to help young women realize a new body-image: that which belongs to the mature woman, not the child.

There are many pressures from society when a girl enters puberty, and she may feel in conflict about her role. But, with education, love, and support a young woman can learn how to move through the physical, spiritual, and sexual transformations of her cycle, without fear, shame or taboo, and with full knowledge of her fertility.

There are ways in which a mother and father can empower their daughter during her first menstruation. The key ingredient is open communication. A mother must speak from her own experience, as teenagers are extremely sensitive to untruths, and a young woman may feel confused if she is told that her periods are "a blessing" and then witnesses her mother's pre-menstrual rage. A mother must come to terms with her own puberty experiences in order to identify with her daughter's.

If you are a mother of a teenage girl, write down your first menstruation experience and share with your daughter what occurred, what was missing for you, and how you believe this may have contributed to your current menstrual experiences.

Ask yourself how old you were when you first started bleeding, did you feel prepared, did you have any discomfort, who did you tell? Were your parents and family members supportive, and how did you feel about this experience? Did anyone explain fertility to you, and how

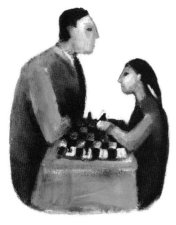

Fathers and daughters

*A father and adolescent daugh-
ter should continue the close
relationship set up in childhood
– while understanding and
acknowledging the sexual
boundaries that should not be
crossed.*

do you feel talking to your own daughter about this?
Finally, ask yourself what you would like to change about
your first menstrual experience and what would have been
the perfect first period for you.

The healing of your own first menstrual experience will
help you to empower your daughter, and end the silence
and shame that so often surrounds the subject of menstruation and fertility.

One of the tragic results of this silence and shame is that
of unwanted teen pregnancies. Without a clear understanding of their reproductive cycle many young women engage
in sexual activities haphazardly. North America has the
highest teen abortion rate in the world.

Most young women begin releasing fertile mucus long
before their first period, and often find this alarming, but as
a mother who understands the cycle and can speak openly,
you will be able to support your daughter in identifying
these changes. You can monitor your own cycle and that of
your daughter's as a non-threatening way of keeping lines
of communication open regarding fertility responsibility
and sexuality. This shared knowledge becomes a tool you
can use to help your daughter become conscious of her
rhythms and to make responsible sexual decisions.

FATHERS AND THE MENARCHE

A father also has a significant role in creating menstrual
wellbeing, because he is the bridge between a young
woman and her future relationships with other men. The
father should continue his intimacy with his daughter
while acknowledging the boundaries that cannot be
crossed during a young woman's sexual maturation. Many
women report how their father grew distant and withdrew,
particularly physically, after they began their periods. The
daughter needs her father to be embracing yet conscious of
the sexually attractive woman who stands before him;
he must be her mentor as "man", yet never partake. This is
the safety the father can invoke as his daughter begins to
experience her sexuality and fertility.

Just as the mother must explore her true feelings about

113

menstruation, the father too must come to terms that his "little girl" has grown up. A father's approval of these subtle changes will increase the daughter's self-esteem and confidence about being a woman.

CELEBRATING THE FIRST BLEEDING TIME

Perhaps one of the reasons contemporary mothers do not celebrate their daughter's menarche is that it marks their own approach to menopause and ageing, and this might be difficult for the mother who fears becoming old and "unattractive". By celebrating and ritualizing the menarche, and initiating your daughter into womanhood, you can become the girl's spiritual gynaecologist: someone who gives her the first experience of body-consciousness. The aim should be to celebrate the spiritual aspects of womanhood, that will enable the young woman to feel positive about her new status as an adult. A celebration of menarche seeks to counterbalance the negativity that still surrounds this event. With ritual, joy, and understanding, you can celebrate the time of the first bleeding as a wonderful and powerful creative awakening, instead of a time of embarrassment or fear.

We can now only imagine the rituals and celebrations of past eras, and so we need to create our own celebrations to reflect contemporary society, and the individuality of every daughter. There are many ways in which you could celebrate (see box, right).

THE MENOPAUSE

The menopause is perhaps one of the most challenging transitions in a woman's life. Unfortunately, it is difficult to welcome the advent of menopause when women are often warned to expect the worst, with symptoms ranging from hot flushes (flashes), to thinning of the vaginal tissues, osteoporosis, and sometimes even psychological disturbances and depression.

In most women the menopause occurs between 48 and 54 years of age, but there is wide variation. For example, surgically induced menopause (the surgical removal of a woman's ovaries) can occur in a woman as young as 22.

Ideas to celebrate the menarche

• A journey, to symbolize going from one maturation point to another, such as a trip to the ocean or the countryside, will enhance your daughter's journey to sexual maturity.

•A gift to mark the rite of passage, whether new clothes, jewellery, or flowers

• A blank book to be used as a menstrual journal

• A special necklace made by you, the mother, and female friends, and relatives

• A patchwork quilt, started on the first bleeding day, in patterns and colours that express your experience of womanhood

• As part of the celebration you could invite your daughter to light a red candle in a peaceful place, and burn some fragrant joss-sticks or incense cones to reflect on the life-giving and creative forces of Nature

The symptoms that herald its onset are usually irregularities in the menstrual cycle, caused by the hormonal changes that are occurring. During menopause the pituitary gland signals to the ovaries to produce less estrogen, and menopause is considered to be complete when there has been no sign of menstruation for two years. Regrettably, in the West – and particularly in the USA – the menopause has become synonymous with hysterectomy. While this surgery may be appropriate for tumours of the reproductive organs, in too many cases it is performed for benign growths, and sometimes in young women of child-bearing age. While it is important that any gynaecological symptom occurring after the menopause should always be explored, it should be with the knowledge and understanding that a hysterectomy does not have to be "inevitable after menopause".

In traditional Chinese medicine, the menopause is seen as one of life's many transitions, with the role of the doctor primarily to help open the gateway. How a woman walks through will vary on the deeply personal nature of the change, and any negativity that surrounds it. In the West, youth and beauty are often valued more than old age, a concept reinforced by advertising and the media, and rarely balanced by images of the wisdom and tranquillity that age and experience foster. No wonder that many women feel anxious about approaching the menopause. As their youthful attributes fade, and their fertility ends, they are apprehensive about a loss of status in a society that values youth, beauty, and fecundity over ageing and wisdom. By contrast, men are considered generally to gain value and attractiveness with age (as in the archetype of the wise old man). Perhaps this is because in Western culture men tend to gain money and power with age, which try as we might, still elude most women.

In cultures where older women gain increased status by becoming the head of the family, menopausal problems are much less common, which indicates that factors other

"The culmination of this skill – the ability to integrate monthly wisdom – peaks at menopause. If women have been successful at listening inwardly each month, menopause becomes the point of power for this developed skill."
TAMARA SLAYTON,
RECLAIMING THE MENSTRUAL MATRIX: EVOLVING FEMININE WISDOM

than hormonal changes are involved. Everything is so interrelated and many factors are influential.

The spiritual aspects of the menstrual cycle – rebirth, oneness with the Earth, cleansing – are rituals in themselves, which is why many menopausal women feel a sense of loss when their periods end. Periods bring a sense of assurance that all is well within one's body, and without them one can feel out of sync with the whole world. Many women, however, find that their monthly body rhythm continues for some years after their actual periods stop, and it is very comforting to know that a cycle can "continue" after menopause.

The more in tune you are with your body, cycle, and emotions, the more likely you are to have an easier menopause. A woman who has learned to value the bleeding as much as the ovulatory side, who has been able to foster good images of herself either mentally or in dreams, is less likely to experience severe menopausal problems.

If you think of the menopause as "late summer", when the leaves are beginning to turn gold, then you will see that it is simply another of life's seasons. Although hormonal changes are inevitable, it is often a woman's fear of the unknown that can bring about the much-feared neurotic state or painful symptoms. Like PMS, menopausal distress may be the result of a society that represses and undervalues the feminine experience and wisdom a woman of this age possesses.

During the menopause you may feel depressed, worthless, and hopeless. Even though you may no longer consciously wish to have a child, the sadness that this option is no longer open to you may be deeply felt. However, if you are in touch with these feelings, if you can share them with others, and allow your emotions space to be, you are less likely to express your sadness in physical symptoms. There is a new freedom in the menopause, since there is no fear of pregnancy.

The expression "change of life" indicates that the menopause does not spell the end of life, but a change of

"There are physical changes in a woman's body during the menopause. If she can accept this and flow with her natural rhythm, if she can accept that there are natural laws and a rhythm to life that we cannot control, then the transition will be much easier."
LYNN OSBORNE

"I felt as if it was the end of my life. My children had left home, and my husband and I were like strangers. I didn't see any point to anything."
ELLEN

Menopausal issues to discuss or to reflect upon
• *Your earliest images, thoughts, and feelings about older women*
• *The elderly women in your childhood/adolescence, and how you felt about them*
• *Your feelings about older women now*
• *Your mother's menopause*
• *Whether you look/looked forward to your menopause*
• *Your understanding of and feelings about Hormone Replacement Therapy (HRT) and hysterectomy*
• *Whether you can imagine menopause as a time of increased vitality, wisdom, and insight*
• *Sharing what would be your perfect menopausal experience*
• *Through understanding the link between menarche, menstruation, and menopause your partner will be more able to support you with love during this transition*

direction. The change can mean an enormous release of energy for some new venture in a new direction, but women who can find no outlet for either their sadness or their experience, can suffer deeply. If you are loved, supported, and helped to understand your emotions, the time of your menopause can be a time for your wisdom to unfold, in which you become more aware of the depths of your own psyche.

In order to recover the power of this stage in life, it helps if women can come together to share the experience of menopause, and to work with their fears about growing old, being alone, unloved, and ignored. Sharing, grieving for the loss of menstruation, and creating a ceremony for initiation will help transform fears into positive power.

WAYS TO EASE THE MENOPAUSAL TRANSITION

• Eat nutritious food
• Start a new activity that will refresh and invigorate you (mental or physical)
• Increase rest and introspection to build up reserves of creative energy
• Awareness of breath, thoughts, feelings, and body through the practice of yoga and meditation
• In some countries, notably the USA, women collectively create a special patchwork quilt. This celebrates, for example, the menarche, marriage, the birth of a first baby, and the menopause. You can start a patchwork quilt as you approach menopause, using patterns and colours that express your own experience of womanhood, and your expectations of the new direction to come
• Sharing feelings – both positive and negative – with other women about the menopause and the changes that it has brought to your life

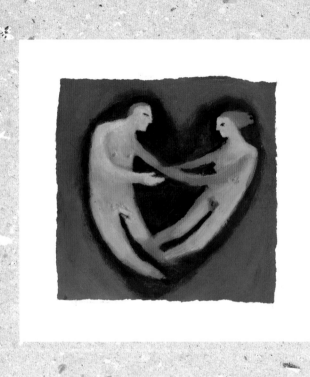

CHAPTER 5

LOVE, SEXUALITY,
AND LOVEMAKING

"The brightness of her cheek would shame those stars,
As day light doth a lamp. . .
See, how she leans her cheek upon her hand!
O, that I were a glove upon that hand.
That I might touch that cheek!"
WILLIAM SHAKESPEARE, *ROMEO AND JULIET*

All human beings have a natural and universal need to be loved, held (see p. 62), and admired, and responded to by others. An infant's survival depends upon a loving and consistent relationship with her/his care-givers. As we develop and mature, our desire for a nurturing relationship generally culminates in the search for a long-term partnership or marriage.

Love is a multi-faceted word, covering many kinds of relationships – friendship, passion, parenthood, partnership (gay and straight), and represents different emotions and diverse experiences. But in every case, being loved begins with loving yourself; not self-centred narcissim or indulgence, but the ability to trust your intuition and listen to your inner voice and heart. Loving yourself may mean recognizing that you are not willing to settle for less than you really want, especially in sexual relationships.

Men and women frequently see love from different perspectives, but beyond that complement, enhance, and inspire each other in unity and healing. Perhaps the confusion lies in our subjective definitions. We cannot define what love is for others.

It is easier to say what love is not. Love does not just happen, or come and go. True love is deep and unconditional and gives of itself. Love is a natural state, it is eternal. Our core and essence is love, and if we allow it, we deeply love our children, our parents, and one another. Strong emotions may need healing if we experience love as being transitory and unpredictable.

Love is not controllable, it simply IS. We can allow it and allow healing to let it through. Love is the most threatening thing to most of us. "I love you" unconditionally said or given makes many of us run; it can completely and utterly threaten our ego. A healthy, undominating ego – a sense of self that does not need to dominate or destroy – requires a healthy early environment, which many of us have not had.

Love is tuning in to your source, and the more you maintain and allow this connection, the more love and loving relationships will manifest themselves around you. It requires trust and courage to let go of the past.

Relationships

The nineties has become the decade of information, with an unprecedented deluge of publications and advice focusing on relationships between women and men. The media and bestselling books such as *Women Who Love Too Much* (1985) by Robin Norwood and *You Just Don't Understand* (1992) by Deborah Tannen reinforce a sense of a frosty war between the sexes, compounding women's feelings of hopelessness about fidelity, relationships, and the lack of available good and loving men as eligible partners.

Woody Allen's movie *Annie Hall* (1975) is considered by many to be the quintessential statement on contemporary relationships between the sexes, perhaps because it sums up the current pessimism people feel about relating to each other. In the closing scene, for example, Woody Allen tells a joke about a man who goes to see a psychiatrist. The man explains that his brother believes he is a chicken. The psychiatrist simply says, "If he thinks he's a chicken, why don't you turn him in?", to which the man replies, "I would, but I need the eggs". As this joke implies, relationships are illogical. They do not make any sense, they often do not work, yet we are compelled to keep seeking them out, "because we need the eggs".

People in so-called "relationships" may live in close proximity, yet have no real "meeting", physically or spiritually. Having respect for the other's privacy is as important as sharing one's thoughts. The deepest communication can very often take place in moments of silence, without the partners having to work directly at the relationship. What matters is to be centred oneself, to be willing and open for the moments of "meeting" when they come. Then the relationship can be trusted to take care of itself. For there to be true relating there must be honesty, love, and the presence of one's true self. It is often our own attitude, not the relationship, on which we need to work.

Most of the time we tend not to relate to each other, because one or both of us is hiding behind screens. We fail to meet one another deeply as we are so seldom in the present moment and "there" for the other person. We seldom listen. There is an inner listening, as well as an outer, which can be learned or ignored.

One of the barriers to relating is that we are often operating on a different level of awareness from the other person. These differences in communication can be called "focused consciousness" – masculine thinking – and "diffuse awareness" – feminine thinking. As masculine and feminine characteristics are so interwoven in both sexes, it is more accurate to speak of these two levels of communicating as qualities that belong to both women and men in varying degrees.

We all use focused consciousness every day of our lives. It helps us to analyse infomation and to formulate ideas; without it there would be no culture, and no medical or scientific advancements. Most children are born with, and many women retain, diffuse awareness. It is related to the wholeness of Nature, where everything is interrelated and

121

where we feel ourselves to be part of a whole.

In general, the basic masculine attitude to life is that of focus, division, and change, whereas diffuse awareness more commonly pertains to feminine thinking. From an early age a girl tends to delight in everything that concerns life and living, while a boy is more likely to show passionate interest in what makes the wheels on his car go round. Women may feel akin to Nature and sense that they are linked to the moon's rhythms; whereas men often want to go to the moon and explore.

Over-awareness of feminine values may paralyse a woman, making action impossible in the outer world. A too focused consciousness in a man may deny the wisdom and intuition from the feminine part of his psyche. Relationships often suffer when these two levels of communicating between the partners become unbalanced and polarized.

INNER WOMAN, INNER MAN

"A man needs to be a man for a woman to be a woman, because you need this constant harmony. If you have a weak man, the woman will tend to take on the masculine, and then she cannot be a woman. It is important for a woman to understand her feminine side, but she also needs some masculine qualities to protect herself in the world on a day-to-day basis. However, if the woman has more masculine qualities than her partner, then the relationship will suffer." Lynn Osborne.

There is no such thing as a simple relationship between one man and one woman. It is always as though many personalities are involved. A happy, healthy relationship requires balance and flow within each of us between the masculine and feminine aspects of our nature.

Each of us has an Inner Man that is associated with active energy, with setting and achieving goals, and with getting things done; and each of us also has an Inner Woman, a natural capacity for letting things happen, for going with the flow of life, relaxing, and being playful. When these feminine and masculine qualities are

Mementos of a love affair
It requires trust and courage consciously to let go of the past, but this is essential in order to allow in new, healthier relationships. Love with another person begins with being able to love and being in touch with yourself. The more you maintain and allow this connection, the more love and loving relationships will evolve around you. Ultimately, we have to find wholeness within ourselves in order to make loving, sustainable, and whole relationships with others.

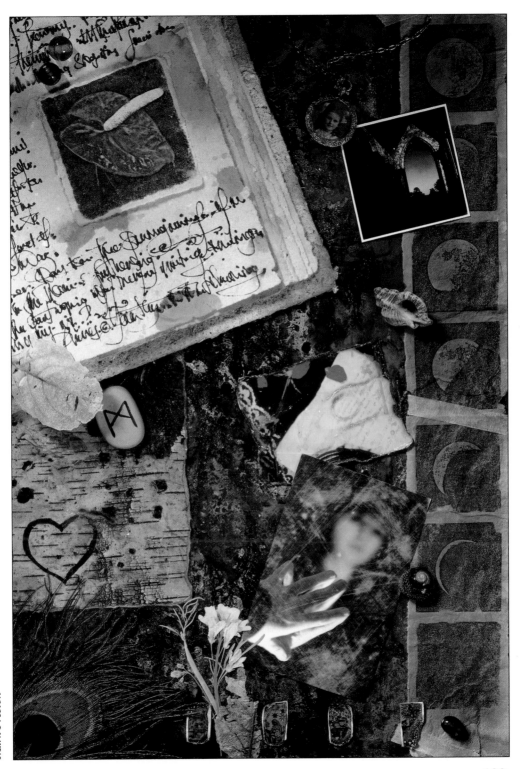

Mark Preston

developed and understood, the union of the two polarities can happen within each person.

While every relationship is unique, we can nevertheless identify common themes and problems, which appear in many intimate partnerships. An individual's imbalances will ultimately affect the quality of his/her relationships and the ability to relate to a partner. For example a man may be so obsessed with his work that he fails to notice his partner and children. He does not communicate his feelings, and denies that anything is wrong. He has unconsciously blocked the feminine side of his psyche, and is too wrapped up in the male world. His behaviour makes his partner feel insecure and increasingly possessive of his outside activities.

Another situation is the woman who is repeatedly drawn to destructive relationships, and who allows herself to be abused and used by men. Her relationship to her animus (her masculine side) is undeveloped, perhaps because of a poor relationship with her father, which has left her unable to protect her femininity.

A third example is the married man who continually indulges in affairs. He believes his wife and children belong in one compartment of his life, and his extra-marital liaisons belong in another. He lacks a strong and solid sense of his male sexuality and attractiveness. This insecurity is reflected in his need for the admiration and excitement of different women; he pretends to be available, and undervalues the women around him.

THE ORIGINS OF RELATING

Our parents' unconditional love and support helps to transmit messages that we are loved for ourselves. Negative conditioning and constant criticism, however, can imprint messages that can lead to feelings of worthlessness and poor self-esteem. A parent is, in this sense, a child's first hypnotist and can give the child either positive or negative suggestions.

In order to reveal and heal emotional wounds so that you can create a loving partnership with another person,

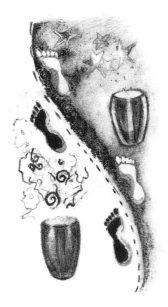

Celebratory traditions

A rite of passage is one of life's important transitions and it can mark the beginning of a profound change. Primitive societies celebrate a girl's menarche and a boy's transition into manhood with familial and social ceremonies, which often include ritualized dancing and music.

you need to understand the ways in which your childhood environment failed you, and connect this to the way in which you relate to your current partner.

Recognizing the limitations and failures of your early environment can be a difficult and painful experience. Yet there is hope from recognizing these connections. With love and support from an enlightened doctor or therapist, you can discard the old messages, their imprints, and their consequent diseases. To take responsibility for sustaining your health you need to uncover and re-evaluate the beliefs you have of yourself, especially those so deeply ingrained that they are unconscious and habitual.

Many women, in recognizing and acknowledging their addiction to destructive, dependent, or uncommitted relationships, have been able to link their patterns of behaviour (alcohol or substance abuse, eating disorders, prostitution, or choices of unreliable partners) to a parent, or parental figure, who abused or failed them in some way. For example, statistics show that the majority of prostitutes have been sexually abused earlier in their lives.

For men, the opportunity to express emotional rage and grief is limited. A new movement aimed at rediscovering and redefining a "new masculinity" has recently emerged in North America, led by author Robert Bly. He brings large groups of men together for weekends in the country to help them discover the Wild Man inside (see also p. 67). Bly believes that strengthening the masculine side of a man not only honours the feminine principle, but is also much more likely to allow the man to develop his femininity.

Bly points out that a man's anima (feminine side) is awakened most strongly when he has the opportunity to contact the wild, passionate side of his maleness. Bly draws on ancient male traditions such as dance, drumming, and initiatory celebrations, to allow a man to truly feel what it is to be a man. When a man feels strong in himself, he does not have to prove his masculinity, so it no longer feels threatening for him to become soft, feminine, receptive, and vulnerable.

During Bly's workshop weekends many men, often for the first time, reveal their pain of childhood emotional and sexual abuse, whether they had remote or absent fathers, or painful relationships with women. When all of this is suppressed and hidden, it can hinder a man from forging and sustaining a healthy relationship with his partner and also with his children.

The future of relationships between women and men lies in each being able to relate to the opposite within themselves, without women being swallowed by their masculine, or men by their feminine characteristics. Ultimately, you have to find wholeness within yourself in order to make loving, sustainable, and whole relationships with others.

Sexuality and society

Our mother's sexuality developed within particular constraints and beliefs, so it is understandable that she might transmit to her daughter apprehension about the female body and the power of female sexuality. A mother's feelings about her own body and sexuality are a crucial influence on the way a daughter will come to feel about herself sexually. Our complex cultural attitudes toward women's bodies – that they are sexual, mysterious, dark, and bloody – find a place in each woman's sense of self. It is rare for a mother to greet her daughter's sexuality in a positive, exciting, and celebratory way. Instead we hear of shame and embarrassment, of adolescent restrictions, and warnings that female sexuality is dangerous, unknown, and unmentionable.

"The union of man and woman is like the mating of Heaven and Earth. It is because of their correct meeting that Heaven and Earth last forever. Humans have lost this secret, and have therefore become mortal. By knowing it the Path to immortality is opened."
SHANG-KU-SAN-TAI

Negative social conditioning about sex creates a fear, which is passed from mother to daughter. Such conditioning cripples our spontaneity and our ability to love one another, and instils in many women fears that it will hurt if we open up more fully to love and bodily pleasure. Instead of a deep communion between two people, lovemaking often becomes an encounter where both partners are afraid to express their real needs. Many women believe the only way to gain tenderness and warmth is to be sexual with a man. If a woman is unable to communicate her needs for non-genital, non-penetrative contact it can often leave her feeling sexually used and abused.

SEX AND SPIRITUALITY

Like the breath, sexual union is a bridge between body and soul, and lovemaking is the conscious way to unite love, spirituality, and sex. The desire to unite sexually with another human being may be a reflection of an underlying spiritual need to return to the original source of our being: the oneness, wholeness, and total intimacy we experienced in our mother's womb.

Sex without love, and its sacred element, is rarely satisfying. When the sexual act is considered to be purely a physical, instinctual drive, carried out solely for the sake of pleasure; when it is not loving, spiritual, or sacred; then the experience of sexual union is not held in reverence or respect.

When repressed and abused, sexual energy becomes associated with personal power and the dominance of one gender over another, and deprived of its loving and sacred dimension it eventually results in disrespect, power struggles, disease, rape, prostitution, and other forms of sexual violence. The huge rise of pornography reflects the split between sexuality, love, and spirit. It leads to alienation, abuse, and hopelessness, and denies our true loving natures.

In Western culture sexuality has become directed toward the masculine goal of intercourse and orgasm. As a result, we follow a male-oriented model of hot, thrusting lovemaking that generally lasts a few minutes and ends abruptly. Included in this model is the myth that "liberated" women want hard, aggressive, and fast sexual intercourse, shown so explicitly in many recent Hollywood movies such as *Basic Instinct* (1992) and *Fatal Attraction* (1987). But intercourse is not just a sexual event; it can be expanded to embrace one's body, mind, heart, and spirit.

Most Western books on sexuality focus on technique

"In early traditions women represented pleasure, joy, beauty and sexual love. Sexual love was a manifestation of the spirit, and not of lust or need, but since spirituality and sex became divided, women have not been able to function fully as sexual and creative beings."
LYNN OSBORNE

127

and performance, which can fill you with expectations that actually prevent experience at its fullest. It is your own personal experience that counts, and this cannot be measured against a mythical "norm" or against generalizations. It is your experience alone that you should be encouraged to develop and trust. You might just as well have books on techniques on how to smile! If your heart is open, and you welcome and permit your own sexual delight, pleasure just happens and comes toward the sun, like a flower.

Many people wonder whether they are performing properly or matching up to past lovers. If there is no expectation from either partner then the pressure to perform will lessen, allowing whatever occurs quite naturally between two people to happen spontaneously. Spontaneity requires both partners to be present at each and every moment.

Ways to enhance your sexual relationship
HONEST EXPRESSION AND COMMUNICATION

Couples often stop feeling sexually attracted to one another, despite still being in love. If you are both harbouring resentments accumulated over time, then when you begin to make love you may feel emotionally choked. This has the effect of blocking your sexual flow, and consequently you can lose your desire.

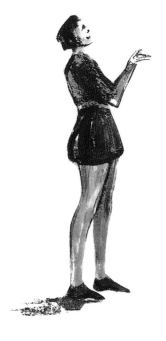

Sexual ecstasy is incompatible with hiding one's feelings. Concealment creates a split in you, which prevents you from wholeheartedly participating in lovemaking. Sharing your fears can heal sexual wounds. The process of exposing and sharing negative feelings – however painful – can often present a great opportunity to expand not only your lovemaking abilities, but your entire relationship with your partner.

You can express suppressed emotion and release past resentment in various ways. Breathing, movement, free expression, massage, and sound, can all assist in releasing blocked emotions and helping the sexual energy to flow.

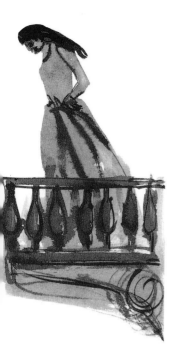

Exchange of love
True love is about give
and take: it is deep and
unconditional, as portrayed
by Shakespeare's characters
Romeo and Juliet.

AWARENESS OF BODY, EMOTIONS, AND BREATHING

Mindfulness (see p. 28) and meditation both form part of sensuality and lovemaking. By being in a position of relaxation and stillness, focusing your attention inside and deepening the rhythm of your breathing, you can quieten the busy chatter of your thought processes. Meditation, which is simply the conscious observation of what is happening inside, can help direct your awareness to your body, heart, and mind during lovemaking. Quietening the mind allows freshness and innocence to return to the act of lovemaking, so that even in a long-term relationship it does not become routine or mechanical.

Spiritual practices speak of the need to surrender, which is another essential aspect of lovemaking. There is much misunderstanding of this term; its meaning is often confused with loss of free will, submission, or with dominance by men over women. But spiritual surrender means to melt into that which is higher than yourself, into love, into spiritual experience It means to open your heart completely, and love and trust your partner.

Many spiritual practices, particularly yoga, place great emphasis on conscious breathing. It energizes body, mind, and spirit and creates an inner silence that allows your sensory perceptions to become much more intense. Being aware of the way you breathe and what it does to your body during lovemaking can help you to connect with your physical sensations, and experience them from within. As you become more sensitive to the flow of your breath you can direct your attention to any part of your body, breathe into that part, create sensations of warmth and aliveness and then spread these to the rest of you. The deeper you breathe, the more you can come into contact with your sexual energy, and the more open your genitals will become, so that pleasure is felt throughout the body.

In lovemaking, as with many intense activities, thoughts often invade the territory of our senses. For example, while making love you may suddenly be distracted by an anxious thought such as, "What if he notices my bulging tummy and post-natal stretch marks?", or, "Am I measuring up to his last lover?" or an extraneous thought about work or other matters may spring from nowhere. Breathing awareness provides a way to free yourself from unwelcome thoughts, and reconnect yourself with your sensations.

You are not judging or pushing the thoughts away, but rather connecting them up with your breath and giving them space to be. Each time a thought distracts you, and you lose awareness of your breathing, notice what happens. Your awareness shifts somewhere else, and your breathing switches back to being shallow and automatic. Moving out of your head and back into your body will come more naturally if you follow the current of your breath, but it does not happen without practice. Be patient and kind to yourself and your partner, and the awareness will come more easily.

HARMONIZING THE INNER WOMAN AND INNER MAN

Just as it is vital for our health and relationships to achieve a balance between the female and male aspects of our nature, so to, during lovemaking both men and women need to have greater awareness of these two polarities.

To integrate your animus (see pp. 20-2) you will need to exercise masculine qualities such as action and assertiveness during lovemaking. Similarly, your partner has to develop his feminine qualities of nurturing and receptivity in order for him to synchronize with your bodily rhythms and peaks of desire.

If your animus is not harmonized, and you have not embraced both polarities, you might sometimes fake your orgasm to protect your partner's self-confidence. However, if you awaken the masculine side of you, you will be able to lovingly, but assertively, tell your partner that you did not reach orgasm and suggest ways in which you both can mutually increase your pleasure.

Similarly, if your partner has not harmonized his feminine side during lovemaking, he may feel uncomfortable when you express yourself during the act. However, if he has awakened his anima, he will be able to enter into love-

"The sexual act requires total surrender on the part of the woman, as she has to completely open herself up. The man has to be able to thrust, so that his penis can reach the tip of her cervix. The man has to be thrusting and active, and the woman open and receptive, and these are the inherent qualities needed in the sexual act. The woman has to melt, and to be able to surrender in this way requires incredible strength. However, because the feminine principle is totally misunderstood, receptivity is rarely seen in this way."
LYNN OSBORNE

making with no preconceived ideas, will be receptive, open to change at any time, and be willing to listen to you.

Biological imagery can help to clarify the ways in which we move between our feminine and masculine principles in our sexual relationships. For example, if your receptive feminine energy is not strong or flexible enough to open yourself to the powerful penetration of masculinity, this can show itself in an inability to allow sexual intercourse. At a basic biological level this is reflected in the failure of the woman to trust her feminine side, and allow her body to let go into full orgasm. The fear of receptivity, as reflected in the condition vaginismus, also is also manifested in emotional blocks that restrict dialogue in daily encounters.

When you are free from stereotypical roles of masculinity and femininity, you are more able to recognize both the male and female aspects of your personality, express them in your lovemaking, and deepen your sexual experiences.

LOVEMAKING AND THE MENSTRUAL CYCLE

When a woman is really in touch with her natural rhythms and accompanying emotions, she knows when she wants to reach out for a hug or cuddle, when she wants to be intimately touched, or when she wishes to become pregnant, and can communicate these differing needs to her partner.

A couple's sex life can be enriched if the man also develops an intuitive understanding of what is happening in his partner. If a woman senses her partner's awareness and deep respect of her femininity, then they will be able to enhance and deepen their lovemaking.

Through intimate knowledge of her inner and outer life, a woman is more able to be more honest about when she does, or does not, want sex. Through fertility awareness (see pp. 84-9) and communication, she and her partner will also be able to discuss openly their desire for a child. In this way, the lovemaking that occurs between the woman and her partner will be more of a real meeting of the spirit.

AWAKENING THE LOVER WITHIN

Discover the potential within yourself – the essential part of you that is already whole, and capable of experiencing

"If a woman can surrender to a man in a totally feminine way, it brings her to a kind of stillness and spiritual strength. This is life-altering for them both, as it totally enhances the man's masculinity."
LYNN OSBORNE

the fullness of sexual pleasure. Instead of looking outside for "Mr Right" to give you the multiple orgasm, you first give to yourself everything that you would give to your beloved. It is liberating and exciting to recognize that you hold within you your sexual destiny.

Loving yourself in this way does not mean selfishly disregarding others, but rather welcoming yourself as the most honoured guest in your own heart. An inner love is a feeling that you can recognize in moments of joy or stillness when deep inside yourself you connect with a natural innocence, simplicity, and spontaneity. This is expressed in your ability to simply be as you are, without trying to be something or someone else.

Part of the process of loving yourself is learning to love your body, through massage, exercise, and making love with yourself. Masturbation is a word with very negative and punitive connotations, but it is simply about giving yourself pleasure. Explore your body as an intimate friend who is accepted, loved, cared for, and cherished, regardless of age, appearance, or shape. If we cannot love our bodies, how are we going to find someone else to love them?

Masturbation is the best way to discover what stimulates you and to show your partner how to please you. Pleasuring yourself can vary, from gentle caresses to your vaginal area during bathing to much stronger dynamic stimulation. The aim need not be to reach orgasm, but simply to explore the sensations. Begin by touching and stroking the inner and outer vaginal lips and surrounding area, varying the pressure and rhythm. It may help to use a natural lubricant such as almond oil. Gently explore the highly sensitive clitoris, and try experiementing with indirect stimulation. Over time, pleasuring yourself in this way, without anxiety or guilt, will increase your ability to become aroused, either with or without a partner.

SACRED MOMENT, SACRED SPACE

The ritual of creating a sacred space or sanctuary for lovemaking will help you to transform your lovemaking into a special and sacred act. A sacred space helps bring greater

132

awareness to the way we think, feel, speak, and experience pleasure during lovemaking.

The chosen room or space where you feel comfortable and undisturbed may be decorated with objects of your choice, such as flowers and candles, beautiful pictures, sculptures, drapes, and incense.

DEEPENING YOUR AWARENESS OF EVERYDAY SENSUALITY

Ecstatic lovemaking can transform the whole of your life, because self-love and spontaneity, pleasure and relaxation, are attitudes you can apply to every area of your life.

Sensuality and awareness can include not just your lover but also your family and environment. The enjoyment you experience during lovemaking need not be an isolated event, unconnected to the rest of your life. You can equally feel sensual and vibrantly alive while listening to a beautiful piece of music, walking down the street, playing with your children, or enjoying good food and wine.

Most practices that enhance sexual intimacy, such as honest communication, meditation, and breathing and body awareness, involve opening the heart to increase your loving feelings and sensitivity – qualities that are bound to affect those close to you.

Deeper sexual intimacy will give you a clearer idea of what nourishes you, and this will encourage you to choose work that helps you to grow and flourish. Creating a sacred space for lovemaking highlights the importance of adding quality time to other areas of your life.

Whenever you find satisfaction, feel it, deepen it, and remember it. This does not necessarily have to include just sexual experiences. Drinking fresh, cool water when you are extremely thirsty, meeting your partner after a long absence, taking a walk along the beach during a beautiful sunset, practising yoga, celebrating close friendships. All of these can cultivate your awareness of pleasurable moments. This will give you the opportunity to expand the joy in your life and can help to break the habit of the mind to focus on problems rather than pleasure.

Remember, there is no "right" or "wrong" way to make

"Images of sex would be better portrayed in terms of poetry, dreams and art, rather than technique. This is much more likely to convey the deep, inner transformative qualities of lovemaking, and the fact that there is an aliveness that you can connect to through your sexual being with your partner."
LYNN OSBORNE

love. You will find your own way, and whatever happens most easily, most spontaneously, and most naturally is "right" for you and your partner.

RESTORING SPIRIT TO SEX THERAPY

Since most sexual conflicts arise from a split between mind, body and spirit, emphasis in sex therapy should be on restoring links between sexuality and the rest of one's life.

Perhaps there are parallels between a woman's sexual behaviour and her general attitudes. For example, if we rush orgasm, what else do we rush in our life? If we push our body in sex, how else do we push ourself? If we find it hard to say "no" in sex, how hard do we find it to say 'no' in the rest of our life?

Integrating sexuality with the other areas of your life helps sex to become less separate and shows how it is another area of living in which many of your familiar patterns and behaviours appear. This does not mean becoming obsessed with sex, but rather that the sexual dimension of our experience is available to us more of the time and is more on a par with other parts of your personality.

Referring to our genitals with beautiful names such as those used in Taoist and Chinese erotic literature may not be appropriate in the clinical settings of Western sexual therapy and gynaecology and in society as a whole. Perhaps this is because words such as "yoni", "lotus", and "jade gate" evoke truly erotic images, where one is fully open and blossoming. All these names are about flowering, closing, opening – a constant flow – and they bring into question the need for a clinical examination of sexuality.

Is it not tension in our body, emotions, and breath that causes problems to develop? If people's hearts feel open, then it follows that their sexual organs will feel more open, receptive, and free.

SEX THERAPY AND WATER

Michel Odent was the first doctor in the West to offer the use of a pool to labouring women to relax and ease the pain of contractions. As his patients began to open up vaginally and allow themselves, physically and emotionally, to sur-

The power of water
The effects of the environment on episodes in a couple's sexual life can be expressed in water metaphors, from the romantic lake during seduction, to the rhythmic waves of orgasm during lovemaking, and contractions during labour.

Myths and legends testify to the irresistible erotic power of water. Honeymooners tend to be attracted to "watery" places, and associating water with eroticism is one of the most common ways advertising agencies promote products, even those that have nothing to do with water.

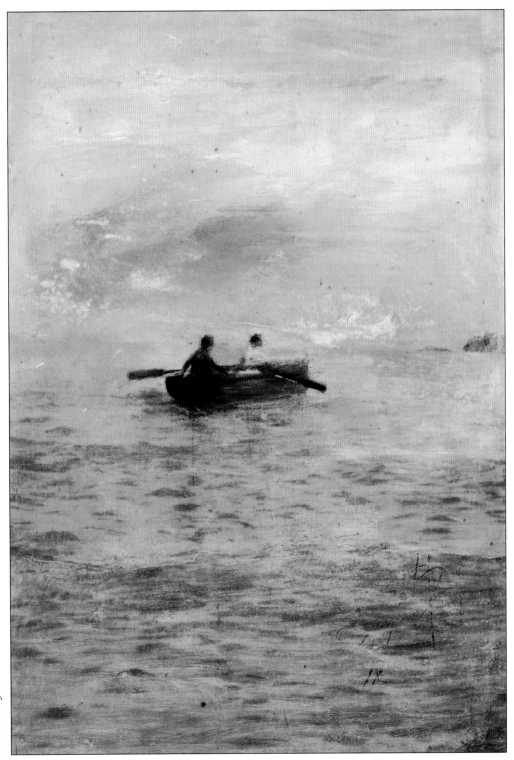

Danielle Blyde

render totally during labour, it confirmed to him that water should also be utilized in sexual therapy. He questioned why there has been such a lack of attention to water in sex therapy, when the therapeutic power of water has been long-acknowledged.

Odent first recognized the important – yet overlooked – role that water can play in healing sexual problems, when a woman came to his clinic and consulted him about her partner's sexual impotence, the cessation of her periods, and their longing for a child. Odent invited her to visit his maternity department, thinking the pregnant mothers and newborn babies would have a positive psychological effect on her. However, to Odent's surprise she was far more interested in the pool in the birthing room, and it occurred to him, that she and her lover should be offered private use of the pool one night.

Some days later the woman contacted Odent to say the idea had been so appealing to them that their sexual desire had suddenly increased, and that her periods had returned. Some months later she called to say she was pregnant.

An holistic sex therapy is one based on healing emotional wounds and trauma rather than simply teaching sexual technique. It affirms that every human being already has within them the natural potential to experience love, wholeness, and fulfilment. According to Odent a sex therapy that does not recognize emotional and spiritual issues, and only concerns itself with technicalities, is not a true therapy.

RHYTHMIC BREATHING WITH A PARTNER

All expressions of rhythm in our lives – particularly lovemaking – are connected with breathing. Learning to use breath as a point of contact between yourself and another person can help to achieve balance, flow, and communication between you.

• Create your sacred space for lovemaking, perhaps light a candle and some incense. Sit facing each other in a comfortable, relaxed position. If it feels more comfortable, close your eyes

• Hold hands, and allow a rhythm of breathing to develop between the two of you

• Breathe in. Breathe out. You're moving into your higher self. Fullness. Emptiness. One follows the other

• Watch the breath flow in, flow out. One blends into the other

• You breathe in. I breathe out. I breathe in. You breathe out. One blends into the other

• The energy fields begin to balance. We are two, yet we are one. Where I stop, you begin. Where do I stop and you begin?

• You are me, I am you, yet I am me and you are you. Blending

• Breathe in. Breathe out. Feelings come. Feelings go. Yet here we are. One. Two. Now I am you. Three, four, open the door

• Memories come. Memories go. And we're here breathing together. Being together. What we've put in is now coming out. And we're here. Learning together. Right here. And now

• Just breathe together. See what happens. Follow it through. Take at least 15 minutes and let nothing else matter

• You may feel your sexual energy rise. Remember that all energy is sexual; all energy is creative. If you decide to make love, explore the energy during the process. Just keep noticing the flow of energy through your body

• Afterward, notice what feelings and thoughts come up during this practice, and discuss them with each other

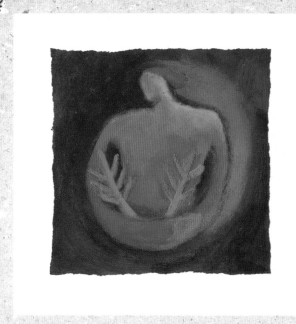

CHAPTER 6

YOU AND YOUR
HEALTH PRACTITIONER

*"The best physicians are those who can find both the
'masculine' and 'feminine' virtues that exist within their
personalities – the ability to make tough decisions and
yet remain compassionate and caring."*
BERNIE S. SIEGEL, MD, LOVE, MEDICINE AND MIRACLES

The first holistic gynaecologists were women, and they
originated in the time of the matriarchal goddess religions
when the cyclical processes of Nature and women's ability
to give birth were revered.

The relationship between the midwife and the birthing
woman was the first healing partnership. It was one
of trust and equality, in which two equals participated
together to bring life into the world.

As civilization developed, women's knowledge of
obstetrics and gynaecology increased. The early healer was
not only a midwife, but also a birthing coach, gynaecologist, paediatrician, nurse, fertility awareness specialist,
geriatric physician, psychologist, and often a veterinarian.
Her developing knowledge of herbs, bodywork, gem-
stones, reflexology, nutrition, and guided meditation,
passed from mother to daughter, and these were the vital
beginnings of science and of medicine.

Men first began to re-enter the field of women's healing
in Western post-classical Europe in the Middle Ages, when
the Christian church's misogyny against women healers
increased. Women who were trained in the old ways of
healing were seen as competition to the new male doctors,

139

and were outlawed from healing – with the exception of childbirth care. Women's bodies were viewed as evil and unclean, so the male doctors refused to handle most deliveries, and midwifery remained in the hands of women until the French male invention of obstetrical forceps in the seventeenth and eighteenth centuries.

From that time on, the remainder of women's health care passed solely into the hands of men, and so were formed the beginnings of male-centred medicine.

Is twentieth-century medicine in need of treatment?

Medical students (male and female) today rarely participate in classes on healing and love, or on how to talk with patients. In many countries too little attention is given to caring and healing and too much to medicating.

Physicians are trained to think that their job is "doing things to patients", in a mechanical way, to make them better and to save their lives.

The best doctors are often those who have themselves been seriously ill, since they appreciate the value of identifying with a patient, (as portrayed in the movie *The Doctor*, 1991). Throughout their training doctors learn not to empathize with the sick, supposedly to save themselves emotional strain. When they talk in medical jargon about a person as an "interesting case", this attitude further distances them from their patient, who is ill and often frightened. So doctors learn to adopt this standard defence against their own pain and failure. However, the emotional distance hurts both parties: the doctor, to defend against the hurt felt for him- or herself, withdraws often when his/her patient's needs are greatest. Doctors need to be taught a rational concern, which allows the expression of feelings without impairing the ability to make decisions.

While a certain amount of distancing may be essential, for most doctors it goes too far, and frequently the pressure of inhumane hours, intolerable working conditions, and so-called detached concern, eventually squeezes out a doctor's innate compassion.

A panel set up by the Association of American Medical Colleges concluded that technological specialization is driving out the exquisite regard for human needs, essential to the relief of suffering. The main task now facing medical schools is to find ways of fostering the feminine principles of caring, listening, and healing, and many colleges are beginning to include courses in humanistic medicine. While doctors tend to be precise in their beliefs and knowledge, they are rarely in touch with their own feelings.

Increasingly patients today are demanding that their physicians apply psychology and spirituality to medicine. Such an outlook can help a doctor to work with his/her heart, as well as his/her head and hands, and share major decisions with the patient. Such an approach will reward the physician as well as the patient, because a doctor who acts out of love does not "burn out". He or she may get tired physically, but not emotionally.

Medical training focuses solely on disease and pathology. As a result, medical students tend to complete their studies with an understanding of disease, but with little knowledge of health. In 1991, an eminent breast cancer surgeon in the United Kingdom claimed that the reason there has been so little progress in the area of breast cancer is because "so little is known about the healthy breast".

Intuitively, many doctors know that there is a way to go beyond their role as a mechanic, but it may take several years of painful self-growth, and opposition from the medical establishment, before they understand how to do so.

A TIME FOR CHANGE

Some doctors (see box, left) have sought to understand what it is like to live with cancer, or mental illness, or the loss of a baby, or the fear of death, and how hard it is to keep one's integrity with that sort of knowledge and fear. They recognize that a typical physician's response – to hide their pain in the face of failure, despair, and errors – helps no one. Bernie Siegel said, "Just like a minister who feels alone because he never learns to talk to God, a doctor feels

---

The inspired few
Some doctors have courageously stepped out of the traditional role of clinician to become more involved with their patients
• *Bernie Siegel, surgeon, and author of* Love, Medicine and Miracles *(1986), who focuses on healing within*
• *The late R.D. ("Ronnie") Laing, psychiatrist, author, and poet, who communicated with mentally disturbed patients*
• *Elisabeth Kubler-Ross has a sensitive approach to the care of the dying*
• *Peter Barr, an Australian paediatrician who supports families who suffer stillbirths*
• *Oliver Sachs, the neurologist whose sensitive methods were portrayed in the movie* Awakenings *(1991)*
• *Frederick Leboyer, the obstetrician who transformed our perceptions of the infant's birthing experience*

141

alone if he or she never learns to talk with patients".

Siegel had become so disillusioned with medicine that he was on the verge of leaving the profession. However, he kept a journal of his feelings, primarily as an outlet for his despair, and through this it dawned on him that he could turn the situation around and still remain a doctor.

The first change he made was to move his desk so that he and his patients faced each other as equals, and he encouraged them to call him by his first name. He discovered that this was an effective way to break down the barriers. It meant he could truly "meet" the other as a person, not in their designated roles of "doctor" and "patient", but as one human being to another.

But moving his desk, and working on a first-name basis, were only symptoms of a larger change. He no longer shielded himself emotionally from the sadness and pain that he witnessed each day, and soon he found he could draw strength, not despair, from his patients. He sometimes hugged them, believing this was because they needed his reassurance, but as time passed he found that he needed to hug them, so that he could go on. Siegel concluded that his only real reason to stay a physician was to offer people a friendship they can feel, just when they need it most.

It occurred to him that medicine had been studying its failures, when it should have been learning from its successes, and he began to see how reliance on statistics had limited his own thinking. Many physicians consider cases of self-healing in cancer patients too mystical to submit to a medical journal, or think that they do not apply to the rest of their patients, which is why most self-induced cures rarely appear in medical literature. Publicizing such cases would help doctors look for them among their own patients and see that healing is not a coincidence. When reversal of a tumour is defined as "spontaneous remission" it teaches doctors nothing about the body's innate healing powers, and stimulates no inquiry into the causes behind the reversal. Bernie Siegel stresses that healing is a creative and dynamic act, calling for the hard work and dedication that any creative act requires of an individual.

Green medicine

The Green Movement heralds a new age of consciousness: an awareness of the importance of our relationships with the environment, with our fellow human beings, and with our inner selves. The role of medicine seems to be developing in isolation from this mood.

In *The Greening of Medicine*, (1990) Patrick Pietroni evocatively describes what it was like to be a junior hospital doctor in London during the "swinging" sixties. He recalls how one night he was helping a famous heart surgeon perform a heart transplant, and the next night, with equal drama and the same amount of adrenaline flowing through his veins, he was listening to the Beatles live.

Both events were the forerunners of changes within medicine and society. The first was an example of the "heroic surgeon" phenomenon, which laid the groundwork for the technological advances of live transplants, in-vitro fertilization, and genetic engineering

The Beatles were an example of another form of breakthrough – that of music, love, ideas, and feelings that were to unite the world. Medical progress in the second half of this century has largely ignored this second breakthrough and has developed in isolation of the feminine world of ideas and feelings. Medicine today is a far cry from the humanist tradition, so steeped in the world of ideas and feelings, from which its study first arose. The world moves on, embracing ecological and spiritual values, and medicine is in danger of being left behind.

Medical advances have to take place not only in the masculine world of technology, but also in the feminine world of ideas and feelings – a revolution in thinking best described by Patrick Pietroni's term "the Greening of medicine". This approach is not "anti-doctor", since its primary aim is to help steer medicine back to its true path.

As the commercial giants now clamour to adopt a "green"

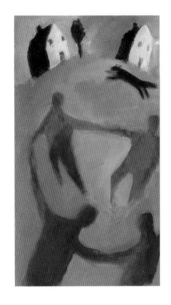

A healthy environment?
Fundamental to good mental and physical health is a healthy environment and the mutual support of community life. People need clean air and water, good food, adequate housing and clothing, and a connection with Nature, which is all too often lacking in today's high-rise developments and crowded inner cities.

143

image, the medical profession is being forced by the public to respond more sensitively to questions concerning health. Unfortunately, this is done in name only. Green issues are health issues, because at every level they impinge upon the quality of our lives, the environments in which we live, and how we relate to each other and to other species. The principles of harmony, balance, and flow, the inter-connectedness of natural phenomena, and the search for inner awareness will form a vital part of the revolution in twenty-first century medicine.

Rather than search for the causes as to why the universe is as it is, the greening process looks for the connections that make the universe as it is. It is a shift from cause to connectedness. In gynaecological terms, this would mean rather than looking for the causes of ovarian cysts, endometriosis, and cancers, the focus would be on under-standing the emotional and physical circumstances in which the dis-eases develop, and the effects and implica-tions on the woman and her immediate relationships.

Patrick Pietroni sees the greening process within medi-cine as the acceptance of limits, the sharing of power, the demystification of the professional expert, and the emer-gence of the consumer interest group.

ENVIRONMENT AND HEALTH

Our early psychological environment can affect our health, and so too can our physical surroundings. The impact of the environment on a person's health is not solely a twenti-eth century, Western concern. Living in harmony with the laws of Nature was one of Hippocrates' basic principles of good health, and his treatise (*circa* 500 BC) on airs, waters, and places (see box, right) is identical in approach to that of an holistic and traditional Chinese doctor's today.

A healthy environment requires love, loving relation-ships, sunlight, clean air and water, adequate housing and clothing, healthy food, and a strong sense of community with family and neighbours, together with opportunity for expression, art, music, song, dance, and a connection with Nature. We have come a long way from this. Instead, we

Hippocrates' treatise
Physicians were advised by Hippocrates to consider the following when treating a patient:
- *The seasons of the year*
- *The winds, both prevail-ing and local*
- *The orientation of the city a person inhabits, in relation to the rising sun*
- *The waters and the ground*
- *Patients' lifestyles: what their pursuits are, and how much they eat and drink*

144

have: air pollution, CFCs and the destruction of the ozone layer, nuclear radiation, water pollution, acid rain, poverty, wars, economic instability, and gross inequality. It is our shame that all this is allowed to go on, when we remember that we are all connected to each other.

The environmental influence on health has largely been ignored by medicine. It has been environmentalists and ecologists, not doctors, who have pointed out the links and the dangers. If we are to understand the relationship between dis-ease and ecological destabilization, the medical profession will need to involve itself more directly in environmental matters. Many modern diseases such as cancer, heart disease, infertility, and arthritis are partly related to environmental problems; what we need is direct action on improving these, rather than pouring research money into high-status specialties such as heart surgery, transplantation, and genetic engineering.

The ambience of the clinical environment and its links with Nature can also influence the health of doctor and patient. In *Love, Medicine and Miracles* (1986), Bernie Siegel explains that when hospital planners removed the windows from operating theatres to improve hygiene, surgeons lost an important source of strength: a connection to God and Nature. A view of the outside world can remind the surgical team of their link to life and Nature. To re-establish this connection, Siegel and an increasing number of surgeons have introduced calming music into the operating room.

GYN-ECOLOGY

"Feel your female planetary body, now, for this moment, and you can sense the pain of our Planet in technological devastation."
TAMARA SLAYTON, *THE ECOLOGY OF BEING FEMALE*

Since the Earth is culturally defined as feminine, we could use an analogy between the condition of the planet and the condition of the female body. They can be thought of metaphorically, and literally, as one and the same. When a woman alienates herself from her "feminine ecology" – fertility awareness, menstruation, and emotions – it can be likened to the crisis of the Earth, which has also become alienated from its own cyclical nature.

A culture that values logic and intervention applies these

145

masculine values to the control of both women and Nature, who are equally seen as threatening, unpredictable, and uncontrollable. Like a woman's body, the Earth becomes something to be owned and controlled.

The Planet is in crisis, her soil tormented, her streams polluted; similarly, the female body is in crisis, her body tormented, her hormonal fluctuations contaminated (by over-use of the Pill, by Hormone Replacement Therapy, and by unnecessary surgery). The values that society imposes on Nature are also imposed on women. Nutritionally, many women are starved of foods that nurture and feed their fertility, and the increasing demands upon women's bodies and the decreasing quality of food continually compromises our health and vitality.

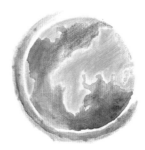

Gaia in crisis
The Earth is Gaia – a living, self-regulating, organism – whose health and stability is necessary for the health and stability of humankind.

Feminine (Gyn) Ecology is a reflection of the Earth. Ecological and human healing are the same. The only way to heal the Planet will be when we begin to own and heal our alienation from our feminine rhythms, sexuality, cycles, and menstrual flow. We have a long way to go, since over 10 million women in our culture cannot conceive; up to 90% of women suffer some menstrual or menopausal distress, and cosmetic surgery, hysterectomies, abortions, and clitoridectomies performed in their millions, (more than 80 million women worldwide are estimated to have undergone clitoridectomy – the ritual surgical removal of the clitoris and parts of the labia).

THE RECOVERY PROCESS LIES IN YOUR ABILITY TO:
• Know what day of the cycle you are in (menstrual or fertile, see pp. 80-3) and draw wisdom, strength, and insight from this self-knowledge
• Bleed on to natural, biodegradable materials, to return menstruation to plant life and to soil. (Menstrual products that contain dioxins and are bleached by chlorine pose serious health risks, both to women's bodies and to the environment by polluting the air, the oceans, and marine life.)
• Anticipate menopause as a time of power, insight,

growth, and wisdom

• Transform your image of women – particularly older women – by looking at beautiful, inspiring older women as role-models for yourself

Feminine medicine

Pressure amongst women for information about health issues appears unstoppable: newspapers, magazines, television programmes, self-help books, and the homebirth movement have all increased the availability of medical facts. Critics of high-tech birth, Caesarean section, radical hysterectomies, mastectomies, and clitoridectomies have all found their campaigners among the increasingly knowledgeable lay woman. The Boston Women's Health Book Collective's book *Our Bodies, Ourselves* (first published in 1975) became symbolic of the explosion of knowledge in women's health. Once again, women were taught by other non-medical women how to practise birth control, regulate their periods, alleviate menstrual and menopausal distress, and challenge obstetricians about the way we give birth.

The coercive messages from society about how women should look and behave have also been challenged by the feminist movement. Bestsellers such as *Fat Is A Feminist Issue* (1978) and *Hunger Strike*, (1986) both by Susie Orbach, and *The Beauty Myth* (1990) by Naomi Wolf, illustrate how women's medical treatments stem from cultural and societal views of women and their bodies.

But it is the emergence of feminine – as opposed to feminist – values that is the most important souce of changes that are now occurring within medicine. Militant feminism would be of no benefit to medicine: it can deny the feminine principle as much as male-dominated medicine can. Hostile, harsh, and unloving attitudes should not form part of any health-care approach.

AN EMERGING FEMININE ERA

Conventional medicine – which is perceived by many to be masculine – is gradually loosing popularity. Conventional medicine classifies diseases, gives them names to distinguish them from one another, and makes diagnoses, the implication being that for each disease there is a specific treatment, and that a disease has a life of its own, apart from the person. Disease is an expression of imbalance, and conventional medicine tends to replace one imbalance with another. While this may be acceptable in the short term, it simply suppresses symptoms at the cost of side-effects and can produce the potential for more serious symptoms, creating with drugs many more chronic diseases.

The new emerging medicine is feminine and maternal, a medicine that perceives a unity between the different aspects of dis-ease, and considers the state of imbalance as the body's way of attempting to heal itself.

"The feminine principle in women's health is to understand the rhythm of the feminine body and how it works."
Lynn Osborne

This new medicine would recognize that certain emotional states, such as faith, love, and hope, can protect health, by inhibiting the secretion of hormones that block the most vulnerable metabolic reactions. Equally, emotions that can promote disease are feelings of despair, helplessness, and hopelessness.

A growing number of Western-trained doctors and health workers firmly believe that the time has come not to separate diseases, but to understand what they all have in common. The starting point would be to ensure that our fundamental needs as human beings are understood, acknowledged and – wherever possible – met.

RESTORING BALANCE AND FLOW TO MEDICINE
The masculine principle has become dominant in all areas of health care, even when women are in practice. Society's denial of natural rhythms often forces women doctors to suppress the feminine, in order to rise through the hierarchy of medicine and gain promotion.

The feminine principle is culturally associated with the skills of listening, nurturing, containment, and receptiveness. Its resurgence has led to the introduction of the therapeutic use of touch, massage, relaxation, and meditation, as well as a recognition of the importance of communication and listening skills in health care. The feminine principle is to listen, to wait, and not to intervene unnecessarily. It can inspire new discoveries through intuition and ideas, due to wisdom and insight.

The masculine principle is to diagnose and intervene; it is the capacity to intellectualize, and act with precision, speed, and firmness. A balance between the two principles is essential. A doctor who works only from the feminine principle would be just as damaging as one working solely from the masculine. For example, if a gynaecologist is faced with a woman who has an ectopic pregnancy, then it is absolutely crucial that surgery is performed without unnecessary delay.

Balance could be introduced to treatment when, for example, a woman consults her gynaecologist about premenstrual syndrome. Instead of saying he has little to offer the patient other than hormone therapy, the doctor could first suggest a change in life-style and diet, or a course of counselling, or recommend homeopathy, acupuncture, or some appropriate alternative therapy.

Elaine Heller, holistic and spiritual counsellor and healer, says "It can be exceedingly helpful to find a doctor who can explain your medical situation clearly and is unbiased towards alternative therapies, so you are assisted in your decisions over what type of treatment would be most appropriate."

The masculine mediates the feminine, and vice versa, but it is rare to be in touch with both of these aspects on an equal basis. Career women, who are familiar with operating more from their intellect, often feel quite confused when, for example, they first become pregnant, as their bodies feel out of control. Pregnancy forces them to look anew at themselves, and become more attuned to their femininity. Having faith in the natural process of pregnancy, and allowing labour to happen, and not being afraid to take our power when we need to push during the final stages of labour to deliver the baby, are all aspects of the feminine.

Although men do not have the obvious body-conscious opportunities of menstruation, pregnancy, and childbirth

"In our Doctor-Healer Network workshops I teach doctors how to relax, how to be human "beings" not human "doings", to allow themselves to listen to the inner voice which tells them when something is not right. The intellect is there, it is not being pushed away, and is needed in emergency situations such as life-saving surgery, but not at the expense of ignoring the doctor's own feelings and intuition."
DANIEL J. BENOR, MD

149

they too can make contact with both aspects. They have the opportunity to develop and become aware of their anima (see pp. 20-2) through relationships, especially with women and children, and more conscious activities connected with the spirit, heart, and Nature. Too often feminists and psychologists dismiss the obvious contact men have with their bodies through being born, being alive, through crying, and through feeling, even if our society tries to suppress these aspects.

Restoring balance into medicine is a process of awareness that needs to be introduced into the training of doctors. These principles cannot be forcibly taught to groups of doctors. They can only be restored to individuals, through helping doctors to find ways of experiencing their own feelings. A doctor needs to be encouraged to notice what is going on inside her/himself during a consultation, as well as the facts the patient presents her/him with.

"Each one of my patients expresses their spirituality in so many different ways, it is like expressing the very nature of life. I feel the best thing is for the practitioner to have space and compassion, for the person to be."
PAULINE O'DRISCOLL

Not only does a doctor need an awareness of self, but also an awareness of vulnerability within her/his role. A way of fostering this awareness is for hospitals to provide support groups for doctors and nurses, where they can talk freely about their feelings, fears, hopes, and visions.

An awareness of the subtle differences and complementary aspects of our feeling and intellectual sides can be encouraged from very early on.

Benig Mauger an analytical psychotherapist endeavours to do this with her children. "My daughter is very soft and nurturing, but tends to be timid. I try to encourage her to do things which also express the masculine side of her nature, such as joining groups and organizing activities. Whereas her younger brother is extrovert and quite tough, so in order to nurture the other side of him I encourage him to sit with me and listen to gentle music. This helps him notice how it makes him feel soft and gentle. I also try to convey to him that it is fine for him to cry and show affection, which my daughter has no difficulty with."

Spirituality and health

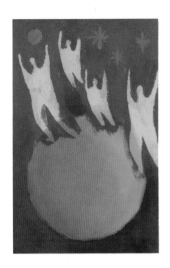

Holistic medicine

"Most illnesses are in some way connected to spiritual dis-ease. Knowing who one is in the universe, and how one functions and why, is vital to health. If a person is unable to manifest herself in this way she will begin to get unwell."
LYNN OSBORNE

People usually consult doctors because they are unwell, but also for human contact, to talk, and to have attention: a kind of confessional. Early medicine and healing was linked strongly to the belief that a person's "spirit" or "soul" formed an integral part of their being. Religion had a major influence in reinforcing the view that mind, spirit, and soul were all closely linked, and helped determine the functioning of the body.

All religious scriptures and spiritual teachings imply that the spirit is more than the sum of emotional and psychological states. The notion of spirit is linked to the concept of a life-force, a transcendent or mystical state of consciousness. Holistic medicine, which sees this energy as integral to its practice, has had no problem integrating spirit into healthcare, as with traditional Chinese medicine's recognition of the life-force of ch'i, and the Indian tradition of the chakras (see pp. 37-44).

Most people's understanding of the human "soul" or "spirit" is "that which lives on after death", and it is this transcendent quality that helps to differentiate spirit from mind. Spirit is often associated with an inner sense of harmony, a knowing from within, and many practices such as meditation and yoga endeavour to encourage the development of these experiences.

Spirituality means something different to each person, and may not necessarily be reflected in any commitment to an organized religion. Spiritual energy is not something that is divorced from the body and which appears only in churches, synagogues, and mosques in response to a God. It is inherent within, and moves physical processes.

Spiritual medicine would include the belief in some meaning in the universe, and would view the force behind creation as a loving, intelligent energy. Some people call this "energy" God, and others see it simply as a source of healing. Spirituality is acceptance of what is. In an ideal world, it is better to make a connection with our spiritual nature before we get ill, rather than to wait until a crisis.

Sickness can often guide us back to the healing connection with our source, which we may have forgotten.

A doctor who is concerned for his patient's spiritual wellbeing is someone who would seek to empower the patient and use what is positive in each patient's beliefs. A "spiritual gynaecologist" would take into account the patient's whole attitude toward relationships with her partner and family, which would give him/her a very much broader picture of her dis-ease. To find out what is wrong with us the doctor asks us – and listens – because s/he knows that listening can be just as healing as "doing". This kind of doctor would not divorce the symptoms from the patient as a person, as this creates a mind-body split. S/he would see the illness as an imbalance within the individual.

Far from being airy and esoteric, spirituality is very basic and down to earth: "After being sterilized, I had symptoms of bleeding and my womb felt on fire. I was put on antibiotics and my gynaecologist suggested a hysterectomy if the symptoms persisted. The healing only finally came about when I was sitting in my garden, and I noticed that my cat was licking her vagina. It suddenly dawned on me that I did not love my body, because how much love does it take to be able to lovingly caress one's vagina and be so in tune?" Mary.

A spiritual gynaecologist would be akin to an earth mother: someone who could help a woman to become more in touch with her body, and enable her to love her womb. A doctor with a knowledge of her/his own psychological processes would be far more able to do this than someone with no inner experience. It is necessary for a doctor to be in touch with her/his own emotional life in order to be receptive to her/his patient's.

One way in which an orthodox/conventional doctor could begin to become more spiritual in her/his work would be to acknowledge that there is a limit to what her/his kind of medicine can do. People can perhaps be more open to change if they admit the limitations of their discipline. If a doctor could allow time to explore her/his own feelings, then a natural awareness and openness, connected to a reverence for life, could unfold.

As doctors and patients begin to understand more about the healing power of love, the spiritual dimension will gradually become integrated into medicine.

WATER, DOLPHINS AND HEALING

In *Water and Sexuality* (1990), Michel Odent uses water and its symbols to illustrate the shift toward a new medical era – an era when treatments will become more broadly therapeutic to the patient, and the role of conventional medicine will be increasingly confined to emergency and life-saving predicaments. He sees our current unprecedented attraction to the use of water in childbirth and healing as evidence of this shift. Water, characterized by yin, is a feminine and maternal symbol. In Hebrew, for example, the word for "feminine" is "nekevah", and the word "nikbah" means water-hole.

Some women are choosing to labour and give birth in water and there is a revival of doctors prescribing treatments in spas. Water is also increasingly being used to help autistic children become socialized.

The uses and power of water are varied and subtle: a blue or turquoise environment can induce a sense of calm, and some rebirthers use immersion in water as a means of deepening the rebirthing experience by mimicking the womb-like relaxed state (see pp. 75-6).

There is a new fascination with the healing potential of the relationship between humans and dolphins. Pregnant women are particularly drawn to dolphins; so too are depressed and introverted people, who have been observed to establish contact immediately with dolphins in the ocean, in a way they have been unable to with humans. The world's first Dolphin Therapy Pool is being developed by Dr. Horace Dobbs in England, to combine dolphin images and sounds with the soothing effect of water.

Whatever we may believe of the dophin theory, the fascination persists. Dolphins seem to have the power to touch us deeply on a physiological and spiritual level – we feel

153

something magical about them. They have a natural playfulness, compassion, intelligence, patience, and the ability to communicate and live peacefully with each other. Stories abound of dolphins saving swimmers from drowning, and of their attempts to communicate with humans, especially those who are vulnerable and ailing.

Maybe the dolphin provides a link with our aquatic past – the time when our ancestors evolved from the sea, and the time we spent in our mother's watery womb. Or perhaps it is simply the dolphins' unconditional love and acceptance of the person beside them that reflects back for us the harmony, joy, and creativity we are trying to re-establish in our lives.

The dolphin symbolizes for us that when people are unconditionally loved and truly in touch with Nature, then they can also find their connection with other life-forms and thereby begin healing themselves and the Planet.

Bridging the gap

The gap between Western (conventional) and alternative medicine should be bridged, not widened further. To use and value only the alternative approach is to dismiss some of the breakthroughs that Western medicine has achieved. We should ideally be looking toward a balance of the two.

Let's assume that Western (conventional) medicine is masculine, directive, and yang, and alternative medicine is feminine, receptive, and yin. Consider the integration of mainstream and alternative medicine as a love story between man and woman, in which the paternalistic orthodoxy meets and becomes infatuated with a more feminine, energy-defined, system. That is, a system that explores the body's subtle energies and healing powers rather than its physical structure (see also pp. 37-44). The feminine medicine in turn is attracted to, and has respect for the history, practical knowledge, and technical expertise of "macho medicine", but is frightened of his mechanistic and material values.

The "dolphin" effect
"Gentle, peaceful and compassionate, [the dolphin] exudes pure happiness and vitality, which suggests a being in perfect mental, physical and spiritual balance".
AMANDA COCHRANE AND KARENA CALLEN, *DOLPHINS AND THEIR POWER TO HEAL*

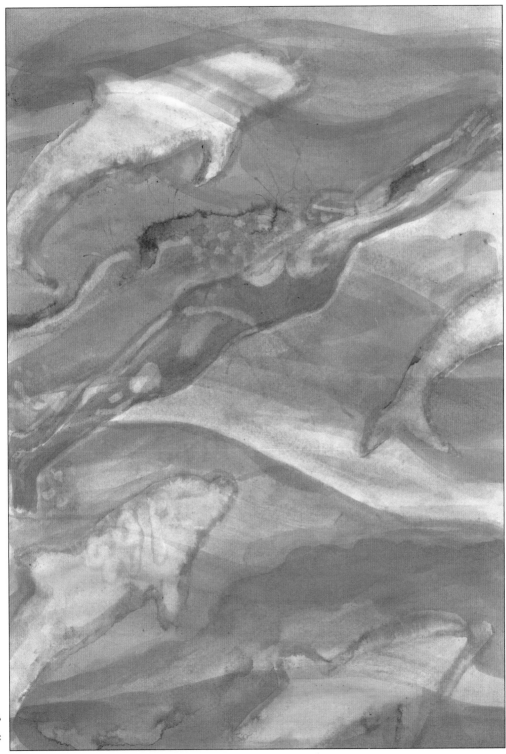

Tiffany Pearson

These different medical models have not yet married. They are still courting, on a part-time basis – as when a general practitioner employs the part-time services of a homeopath, psychotherapist, or acupuncturist, and even this is still very rare. Often they are trying to deny, even to themselves, their involvement with one another. They are both struggling to see whether or not it is possible to reconcile their differences, because they both sense the potential benefits to patients.

"I believe that once a health practitioner evolves beyond the 'medical approach' and allows the possibility of other very real energies being involved in illness and disease, a radical change has occurred in the practitioner."
YOLANDA S. WESTCOTT, MD

Then the couple conceive a "child" – holistic medicine – a union that has properties of both approaches, and is potentially very powerful as an integrated medical model.

The use of the parental analogy (originally proposed by Dorothy Wallstein in *The Homeopath*, September 1990) imaginatively illustrates the issues now facing orthodox doctors and complementary practitioners. Responsibility for their "child's" future, will be in planning for its future together. They both need to recognize the limitations and weaknesses on both sides, and negotiate to form a bridge of common ground. It means that as well as doctors practising in a holistic way, and integrating alternative approaches into their practice, alternative practitioners would have to recognize that orthodox medicine has its place too. The two styles of practice should be complementary to one another, not subservient or competitive.

BUILDING BRIDGES

There is far more common ground between conventional and alternative approaches than might at first be realized. However, in order to bridge this gap, alternative practitioners may be required to explain their approach and translate this into a common language. Such a partnership is more likely to take place when two health workers can work closely alongside one another.

We need all the different forms of medicine to treat the different levels of illnesses, but they need to be integrated. If you break a leg, then you need to have the orthodox treatments such as surgery and manipulation, and also alternative remedies to promote the healing. In cases such as a fracture, concussion, and extreme emergency, conventional (allopathic) medicine is vital and wholly appropriate; it would be inappropriate to simply rely on natural remedies.

Conventional treatments only become inappropriate when they are used without considering whether they are necessary, or when they fail to give a patient choice. For example, the routine removal of tonsils, or the prescription of steroid creams for eczema, are inappropriate treatments when less invasive homeopathic treatments and acupuncture can be more successful. Many people would welcome using these gentler methods if they were given the choice between them and surgery. Alternative treatments are not non-interventionist so much as gentle interventionist. It is important to allow the patient to make an informed choice about what is appropriate and feels right for her/him, whether orthodox (conventional) or alternative treatment. People also need to be helped to understand that they are capable of healing their life more, and that this could also cause their symptoms to disappear.

Alternative therapies tend to encourage more responsibility and consciousness of lifestyle imbalances that lie behind the symptoms. This increased awareness leads the patient to seek professional help swiftly, when symptoms of imbalance or ill health do appear. However, there will always be people who opt for material interventions (surgery/drugs) because they prefer to "get things fixed", or are perhaps frightened to explore what lies behind the symptoms. If, for example, a woman has been bleeding from fibroids for over three years, but only consults her homeopath when she is very ill, and uses the remedies purely as a last resort, it may be appropriate for the homeopath to suggest surgery, since the patient may not be willing, or able, to make fundamental changes to her life.

The formation of the Holistic Medical Associations in the United Kingdom, United States, Canada, and Japan has been a major breakthrough in building bridges between allopathic doctors and complementary practitioners. The

Marylebone Health Centre in London uses homeopathy, traditional Chinese medicine, osteopathy, massage, counselling, and stress management alongside conventional medicine in a National Health Service multidisciplinary team. Furthermore, doctors elsewhere have begun to explore the value of combining alternative therapies with orthodox medicine by introducing aromatherapy, massage, and psychotherapy into their hospitals.

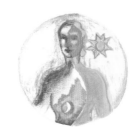

Restoring balance and flow to medicine
Balancing feminine and masculine principles in medicine is a process that needs to be incorporated into the training of all health practitioners.

As consumers of health care we have the power to effect change. The clearer we become about what we want from our doctors and health care, the more we can begin to work with them to realize our vision of better health care.

The relationship with your health practitioner

It is in the medical encounter that many women experience the imbalance of power most personally. In particular, the gynaecologist – as a surgeon – stands at the apex of the medical hierarchy. When we consult her/him we are usually at our most exposed and vulnerable. Although the substance of institutional power needs to change, personal assertiveness will not shift this power differential. While thinking positively, and becoming more aware, may make you feel better, it will not of itself change the structures.

HOW TO FIND AN ALTERNATIVE HEALTH PRACTITIONER
• The safest routes to obtaining an alternative practitioner are generally through personal recommendation, your family doctor, or a recognized organization (see Resources, pp. 210-17)
• Your doctor can also approach the British Holistic Medical Association (BHMA), the Canadian Holistic Medical Association (CHMA), or the American Holistic Medical Association (AHMA), for listings of local practitioners (see Resources, pp. 210-17)
• In the United Kingdom there is a Doctor-Healer Network, which currently consists of five groups around the country. Following their international

conference in October 1992, they hope to expand their network (see Resources, pp. 210-17)

• Trust your own feelings and impressions whether you are searching for a complementary practitioner, or a mainstream medical doctor or a gynaecologist. Ask yourself whether you feel comfortable talking to him or her? Do you trust him/her professionally? Do you feel you are being seen and heard as an individual? Choose someone who shares your awareness. Simply being in the presence of someone may – on an intuitive level – give you a good indication of their professional and personal qualities

• See Resources (pp. 210-17) for an extensive listing of holistic organizations and practitioners

• Many traditional doctors are now becoming more open to working in a complementary way with alternative therapists. Ask what your doctor's opinion is about these therapies and whether he or she has had experience of them

WHAT TO LOOK FOR IN A HEALTH PRACTITIONER

The qualities that patients look for in a practitioner are varied and diverse, and it is often the case that we choose the person, not the treatment. In other words, we are more interested in finding someone with whom a good professional relationship can be established, than in the particular treatment he or she provides.

Just as you would expect an orthodox/conventional doctor to be professionally qualified, expect the same of an alternative health practitioner. As the law stands at present anyone can advertise himself or herself as a psychotherapist or "healer" without specified training, subjection to a code of practice, or inclusion in a central register of practitioners. If a homeopath, hypnotherapist, traditional Chinese doctor, or acupuncturist is a member of an organization it is some guarantee of competence, and can also minimize the risk of exploitation. Also be aware that not all complementary therapies are holistic in their outlook, nor are all conventional (allopathic) doctors un-holistic in their approach to patient care.

Open-mindedness, empathy, and support are the hall-marks of a good physician/health practitioner who is truly committed to helping the patient. A therapist should have integrity, since many issues surrounding women's health are of an intimate and delicate nature, and the fact that a practitioner belongs to an organization means that he or she will be subject to some degree of regulation by colleagues. Skills such as listening, massage, and touch can also be very beneficial. A characteristic of many complementary therapies, which makes them very attractive, is that they give some measure of control back to the patient, empowering and allowing you to regain your self-esteem.

To ensure that you undertake an appropriate course of therapy, seek an initial consultation before committing yourself to any particular approach. This offers you an opportunity to meet with the practitioner or therapist, and to talk over what feels best for you.

PRINCIPLES OF PRACTICE TO LOOK FOR
• The practitioner adopts an holistic approach. That is, he or she responds to your emotional and spiritual needs, as well as your physical symptoms
• She or he ensures that you have the right to assume responsibility for your own health
• She or he is able, and willing, to teach you how to practise life-style changes to help enhance your life and to help prevent diseases from occurring or recurring
• S/he uses, or approves of the use of "safe and gentle" therapies to both counteract disease and enhance your life in general
• S/he is aware of any personal feelings of racism, moral judgement, and sexism that s/he might have, and acknowledges the discriminatory practices within his/her profession
• S/he is sensitive to the cultural taboos that forbid

certain women from being examined by a male doctor and, when necessary, can refer patients to a female gynaecologist instead. (A survey conducted by the Australian Health Service found that fear of moral judgement and undressing in front of male doctors may be stopping Chinese women from having vital cervical smear (Pap) tests, and gynaecological check-ups.)

The practices of psychology and psychotherapy are not immune to imbalance and their practitioners also need to integrate feminine and spiritual values into their approaches by addressing the issues of race, culture, sexism, and poverty, all of which can influence the therapist's view of his client.

Although psychotherapy is sometimes considered "alternative" and a "fringe" medicine, its patients are not immune to intervention and abuse. For example, the power imbalance between male therapists and female patients can be exploited by the therapist, causing danger and abuse, and continue to happen all under the guise of therapy. Negligence, power imbalance, and abuse occur not only in Western medicine, but also in what are often considered "safer" and more "natural" approaches, such as individual and group psychotherapy.

HEALTH RESPONSIBILITY

Physicians are created as much by their patients as by their training. Most people unconsciously want to give up all decisions to a powerful parental figure. You can begin to improve your health only when you realize that you have to make your own decisions. Becoming responsible for your health may require some hard work, which can seem daunting. Consequently, when offered the choice between an operation and a change in lifestyle, some of you will opt for surgery, which may seem easier and less trouble.

In our consumer age we increasingly demand new drugs and miracle cures. The fact that many common ailments could be alleviated by a change of lifestyle and

"Doctors are generally working to the best of their ability, but like all human beings they can't always know everything and always be right."
ELAINE HELLER, HOLISTIC AND SPIRITUAL COUNSELLOR AND HEALER

diet, and increased relaxation and exercise, does not always influence us. It is often easier to place the blame for the causes of most illnesses on external factors.

Taking charge of your life to achieve health and peace of mind will require some effort. Most of us do not make full use of our potential for health until a near-fatal illness, or crisis, forces us to change our lifestyle. But it does not have to be a last-minute awakening; it is best to start becoming conscious of your health before getting sick. The mind's power to heal is available to you all the time, and it has more room to manoeuvre before a serious illness threatens.

To begin this process you need to find that part of yourself that can choose the best advice, and follow it. Transformation does not come from the intellect and rationality; it comes from finding your authentic self, and following what you feel is your own true path in life. You may need a health practitioner (or a yoga group, a supportive family or a friend), who can act as an initial guide.

Becoming more responsible for your health means that you would not rely solely on your doctor to take the initiative, but rather use him or her as a member of a team – of which you yourself are part. Increased responsibility would require you to educate yourself in your own care.

"It could be said that a doctor who is aware of their limitations is the best kind of doctor. It is also becoming more generally accepted by the medical profession that spirituality exists and is a necessary part of the care given to patients – as defined by the World Health Organisation – who stated that health has to include mind, body and spirit."
ELAINE HELLER

HOW TO TAKE CHARGE OF YOUR OWN HEALTH CARE
• Question your doctor so that you understand your treatment
• Use self-assertiveness to create a more effective healing relationship. If you can speak your mind, a healer can better help you
• Question authority, tests, and results. Don't take them for granted: if you are unhappy, seek a second opinion elsewhere
• Speak up for yourself, your needs and comfort in all areas, both before and during examinations
• Make your practitioner aware of your unique needs and desires by discussing issues
• Connect with your feminine side to reach your

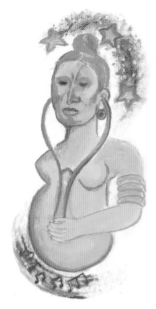

The feminine principle
This is culturally associated with skills of listening, communicating, nurturing, containment, and receptiveness. You can apply the feminine principle to your own health care by listening to and trusting your own body, and by utilizing your body's innate healing potential.

inner feelings, and build your relationship with yourself. If you are faced with a decision about whether to have surgery or seek an alternative approach, then your informed decision has to come from this inner place. However, you may need counselling for negative emotions such as fear, guilt, or denial.

FOSTERING TRUST AND CONFIDENCE

A bond between you and your practitioner comes about largely as a result of your confidence and trust in the healing relationship. Trust can be forged in many ways, but certain essentials usually include openness, compassion, acceptance, honesty, availability, and the practitioner's willingness to provide you with information.

One of the best ways to make something happen is to predict it and believe it will occur! Studies show that one-third of patients will improve if they merely believe they are taking an effective medicine, even if the pill they are taking has no active ingredient (this is known as the "placebo" effect).

• Studies have found that those patients with a high level of trust in their doctors heal faster than other patients. The relationship between you and your practitioner may be as important as any medical or surgical procedure

• To create a relationship of trust, you and your practitioner will need to learn each other's beliefs

• Your practitioner's confidence in a certain treatment can be negated by your unspoken rejection of it. Bernie Siegel encourages his patients to draw and report their dreams to help him to learn about their unacknowledged feelings about certain procedures

• If you do not want a particular procedure from the start, but do not have the courage to tell your doctor, you may reject it at an unconscious level

• If your doctor knows how you perceive a treat-

163

ment, s/he can proceed from that point. S/he may be able to modify your attitude, or choose a different form of therapy.

PREPARING FOR SURGERY

The most common operations performed on women by gynaecologists include hysterectomies, D and Cs (dilation and curettage – the scraping of the womb's lining), removal of fibroids and ovarian cysts, investigative surgery for infertility and unexplained pelvic pain, and pregnancy terminations.

• If you are to undergo surgery, major or minor, a pre-operative visit by your gynaecologist and his/her surgical team is important. This visit will not only help you through the surgery, but can also speed recovery. A study showed that patients who received a visit from the anaesthetist the night before surgery, as well as explanations and reassurances about their surgery, needed only half as much pain medication, and left the hospital two-and-a-half days sooner than a control group of patients who were not talked to or visited

• Take a tape recorder to the hospital, with your favourite music or meditation tapes, if you use them. Ask for them to be played in the operating and recovery rooms, so you can hear them during and after surgery

• Speak to your body, particularly the night before surgery, suggesting to it, and particularly the area of surgery, that your cells will heal rapidly

• If you have to have surgery of any kind, stipulate beforehand that you do not wish to have a vaginal examination (for teaching purposes), while under anaesthetic

• While you are recovering arrange visits and calls from people who you feel love and support you

*"For many women who even-
tually have sex in the forbidden
zone, the wish for connection
originates in the hope for
restoration of a lost father-
daughter (or even
mother-daughter) bond. . . A
woman who feels a reawaken-
ing of hope with a man may
wish to touch him or be
touched by him."*
PETER RUTTER MD, *SEX IN
THE FORBIDDEN ZONE*

PROFESSIONAL ABUSE AND THE ISSUES OF POWER

A doctor, health practitioner, or therapist unconsciously represents a parent or idealized figure when we seek their help, and the hope and trust that we place in them can open the door to abuse.

While the majority of health professionals are trust-worthy, and respect a woman's vulnerability while under their care, cases have been reported of abuse in the clinical relationship through inappropriate sexual behaviour.

Many women feel vulnerable and are unable either to protect themselves, or confront the abuser. There are cases of a woman's breasts being "examined" when a woman consulted an osteopath for a painful knee; and a woman with a skin rash on her leg was asked to remove her bra by a doctor. It may not always be physical abuse: one woman consulted a homeopath who questioned her sex life in such a prurient way that she felt uncomfortable and afterward ashamed, yet paralyzed to stop his questioning.

TYPES OF ABUSE
- Physically touching the patient inappropriately
- Making suggestive comments or requesting the patient to undress when it is clearly unnecessary
- Shouting at her and becoming verbally abusive
- Using the patient as an unwitting "case" example in front of students and humiliating her in public to illustrate a point s/he is trying to make to them
- Entering the patient into a clinical trial without her informed consent
- Removing the patient's womb and/or ovaries during investigative surgery without the woman's informed consent
- Projecting his/her own sexual or moral values and opinions on to her
- Assuming or implying that the patient should be having sex, even if she has chosen celibacy
- Assuming or implying that she should be having sex with someone of the opposite sex

165

If anything in a consultation makes you feel the slightest bit uncomfortable, you should, in the first instance, try to tell the practitioner, to clarify any misunderstandings. If, however, you cannot, or this does not allay your anxieties, you should advise him/her that you consider him/her to have abused his/her position, and that you will be writing to the General Medical Council if s/he is a doctor, or his/her professional organization if s/he is an alternative practitioner. Only by reporting such incidents can women make organizations aware of them, and be able to take appropriate action.

For health practitioners

The patient you might consider the most difficult or uncooperative is often the one who is most highly motivated and most likely to get well. One study in the United States finds that long-term breast cancer survivors were those considered "difficult" by their doctor; who asked a lot of questions and expressed their emotions freely.

If a patient is very insistent in wanting to know the details of her illness, laboratory tests, and treatment, provide her with all the information she needs: this has been shown to improve her wellbeing dramatically.

More than any other factor, participation in the decision-making process determines the quality of the doctor-patient relationship. If a patient wishes to share responsibility for her health and treatment, and you encourage this attitude, it can help her to heal faster.

Create a healing space for your patient, and within that space it is essential that you accept whatever feelings she exposes – be they anger, fear, grief, love – and make the person feel safe. If you can accept the patient as an individual, with choices and equality, options and information, you and she will become a team, working together in the healing process.

COMBINING YOUR BELIEFS – BRIDGING THE GAP

It has been found that a patient's body responds directly to her own beliefs, not her doctor's. This means that even if

Homage to the Earth
Buddhist scriptures see the human body as a reflection of the Earth. They liken our eyes to the sun and moon, which open and close like day and night, our breath to the wind, and our arteries and veins to the streams and rivers. Just as we should love and trust our bodies we should care and love our precious and beautiful Earth. Feminine and planetary healing are inextricably linked.

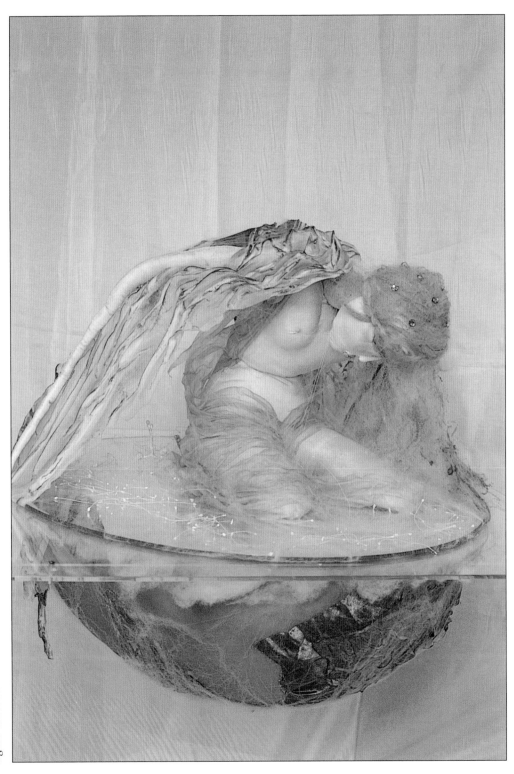

Agnes Chevalier

you and your patient share similar views and beliefs about treatments, ultimately it will be her beliefs that will influence the outcome of the treatment, rather than the doctor's.

If you run out of remedies or solutions for a patient you may feel like giving up. Remember, however, that your lack of faith in a patient's ability to heal can severely limit that ability. Never tell the patient that there is nothing more that can be done for her. There is always something more you can do, even if it is only to sit down, talk, and help reassure her.

While it is your duty to accept all patients, you do not necessarily have to support all their choices. For instance, you have a right to say, "I can't agree with what you're doing, and don't want to participate in it", but usually this ends the healing partnership. Instead you might say, "I don't agree with what you're doing, because I don't think it's the most appropriate treatment, but I will help in any way I can if you wish". Then, if the woman finds that her choice is not productive, she will feel more able to return to you for advice.

Since patients seldom open up to unreceptive doctors, the more open you and your colleagues become, the more your patients will reveal to you, and the more we will all learn. For example, if a patient reports amazing improvements in her health, you may find, if you enquire, that she has made some drastic changes toward a more loving and accepting outlook.

The best results proceed from a negotiation in which your viewpoint and that of your patient come close enough for true communication. If, for example, she fervently believes in homeopathy for her fibroids or heavy periods, then you should not become an obstacle and detract from that treatment's effectiveness. Even if you think such methods are useless, they are likely to help if your patient believes in them.

Try to work to see how your beliefs can combine truly to bridge the gap between conventional/orthodox and complementary medicine. The measure of effective health care

"The experienced reality of the doctor is so different from that of the patient, and the biggest bridging of this gap is not so much in the area of 'what' you are doing, but 'how' you are doing it. Listening is a skill which can be learned and trained – it is an imperative quality, because when the doctor starts to listen he or she begins to make real contact."
RUUD ODERKERK, MD

is how well you and your patient accept each other's beliefs, and are able to translate them into a common language, even though they may differ.

If your patient has no faith in your methods, she will resist treatment consciously or unconsciously, which is bound to thwart the healing process.

Bridging the gap between conventional (allopathic) and alternative gynaecology means that you and your patient need not reject standard medical techniques as an option. Most of us, when faced with a serious illness, are simply not strong enough to heal ourselves completely through finding peace of mind and developing a new awareness. While your patient works to increase her consciousness and change her lifestyle, orthodox treatment such as drugs and surgery can act as a support until she is well enough to rely more on holistic methods.

IN THE OPERATING THEATRE

A doctor's attitude counts, even when a patient is under anaesthesia. Studies confirm that voices known to patients are heard and understood during anaesthesia. Recent work has confirmed this unconscious awareness, whereby anaesthetized patients were played a tape with instructions, with which they promptly complied.

"Surgery can either be a loving, spiritual experience, or it can be like going to a butcher and being treated like meat. What makes the difference is the doctor's awareness of the person who is suffering the illness, rather than the illness the person is suffering from."
DANIEL J. BENOR, MD

In his operating room in New Haven, in the United States, Bernie Siegel constantly communicates with patients about what is happening. And many anaesthetists have begun giving their anaesthetized patients calming messages, and implanting positive thoughts. Surgeons are using the anaesthetized mind's powers to help prevent complications, by for example suggesting to the anaesthetized patient that they will be able to relax crucial muscles afterward.

Try to ensure that your surgical team do not say anything they would not say if your patient were awake, and to avoid negative messages. A simple statement like, "You will wake up comfortable, thirsty, and hungry" has been found to promote recovery. Yogis and hypnotized subjects can control bleeding, and the request to the patient

169

during anaesthesia not to bleed also seems to work. Even if this may seem strange to you at first, there is no reason not to communicate with a patient in every possible way.

The ambience of the operating room can also influence the attitude of both you and the patient. If there is no view of the outside world to remind you of your link to life, one way of re-establishing your connection to nature in the theatre is to use music. Music opens a spiritual window. Its healing properties have been known about since time immemorial, and it can serve to calm both your patient and your staff, helping them deal with stress. Rather than distracting them from the surgery, music should focus everyone's attention on the fact that there is a living person being operated on, and can help your staff relate to that person as though she were awake.

AWARENESS OF COMMUNICATIONS
Empathy can build the connection needed for healing, and because of its effect on the patient, your conscious and unconscious attitudes are often crucial to the success of treatment.

Your patients must feel confident that they have your undivided attention. A surgeon's schedule is often extremely pressured, but if you sit down for one minute at a patient's bedside to talk, your patient is likely to experience it as much longer. If however you simply stand in the doorway, the same visit can seem more like fifteen seconds.

Our minds and bodies communicate constantly with each other, but mostly this is on an unconscious level. Doctors in ancient history, including Hippocrates, were well aware of this, and used the interpretations of their patients' dreams as essential diagnostic and curative tools. Dreams can often give a richness of information that medical tests cannot. Some are easy to interpret, and often you and the patient will be able to understand a dream simply by discussing it together. Today, dream interpretation is a lost art in medicine, reserved purely for psychoanalysis. It is just beginning to be studied again and it is hoped that it will once more become a tool that all doctors can use.

170

Another way to reveal a patient's unconscious beliefs, is through her drawings. You can ask her to draw a picture or image of herself, her treatment, and her symptoms. Such drawings can by-pass verbal deceptions, and reveal the universal symbolic language of the unconscious. Bernie Siegel has found analysis of his patients' drawings to be one of his most accurate aids to prognosis.

The failure of many doctors to interact creatively with patients may come partly from the way they have been taught to be "mechanics", to learn all about disease, but nothing about what the illness means to the sufferer. One way you can begin to understand a patient's experience of her illness is to ask, when appropriate, what she thinks has caused it, what threats, losses, or gains the condition represents to her, and how she believes it should be treated.

The use of dream interpretation, drawings, and open communication are all methods you can use to achieve a greater understanding of, and sensitivity to, your patient's experience of illness. Dreams can also offer a unique chance to reach your own unconscious. For men, your inner feminine self is waiting to be discovered and to be integrated into your medical practice. Through your experience of dreams – as well as those of your patients' – you can begin to understand this feminine side of your nature. All the players in dreams are part of you, your psyche, and your conscious work can be to integrate those sides – including the compassionate feminine – into your psyche and use it to heal yourself and your patients.

PROFESSIONAL ABUSE

The imbalance of power that exists in society between men and women is often recreated in the clinical setting between male doctors and female patients. Although it is a sensitive and taboo issue, professional abuse nevertheless has to be faced in order for it to be healed. The issues of power and ethics in the consulting room are not only confined to gynaecologists but to all health professionals, psychotherapists, and also to teachers, clergy, and lawyers.

Although the vast majority of practitioners practice with integrity and excellence, all health professionals need to become aware and open about their vulnerabilities, temptations, and mistakes. Only through a sharing, non-judgemental forum can problems of abuse be worked through in order to create a healthy model for practitioners and patients.

"It is important to clarify the distinction between forbidden sexual acts and sexual feelings. It is entirely natural to have sexual feelings and fantasies in any relationship of importance. The ability to avoid acting on these feelings is the central challenge of maintaining respect for sexual boundaries." PETER RUTTER MD, SEX IN THE FORBIDDEN ZONE

SOME OF THE ISSUES THAT NEED TO BE EXPLORED
- What constitutes sexual abuse and what does not?
- What makes a health practitioner vulnerable to crossing a boundary?
- When is it acceptable – if ever – to commence an intimate relationship with an ex-patient?
- Health professionals having sexual fantasies about the patient when she is in the consulting room
- Health professionals ignoring, doubting, minimizing, or denying what patients tell them
- Health practitioners playing "therapist" without telling the patient what s/he is doing, and without having the training to do so

A patient with sexual difficulties may not always first approach a sex therapist. The woman may consult a gynaecologist or homeopath, which may require the practitioner to ask the woman intimate details. If it is inappropriate to refer her to a sex therapist, you as her practitioner might begin by first asking yourself:

- Why do you want to delve into this area?
- Is it important or relevant to your prescribing to find out about your patient's sexuality?
- If it is, share your thoughts with the patient. Explain to her why it is relevant and create a safe boundary by assuring her that the consultation is confidential and that nothing that is said will go beyond the room
- Check out your patient's willingness to talk about

her sexuality. If there is even the slightest hesitation, offer her the choice of coming back to it in her own time if she wishes to

• Begin by asking non-threatening questions such as, "Is it OK with you if I ask you some questions about your sex life?", followed by, "Is there anything that is troubling you in your relationship? Are you happy, for example, with your sexual relationship?"

• Whenever sensitive issues are raised or discussed regarding past sexual abuse or current sexual difficulties, you should ensure that the woman's experiences are believed and validated. In other words, the patient must be "heard" at all times

• The tone of your voice, posture, expression, and words should convey at all times that you are trustworthy, non-judgemental, and safe

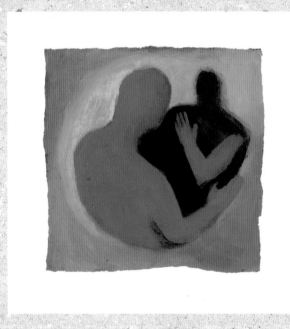

CHAPTER 7

INTIMATE HEALTH, TREATMENT
AND SELF-HELP

*"For a woman, wellness is significantly defined by her
relationship to her menstrual cycle, and her ability to
gather wisdom, direction and insight from the ebb and
flow of her hormonal changes."*
TAMARA SLAYTON,
RECLAIMING THE MENSTRUAL MATRIX

This chapter is about taking responsibility for your own
health and making the most of the treatments available,
both orthodox (conventional) and complementary therapies. Advice and suggestions for treating a number of
health conditions are presented in the second half of the
chapter. First, we discuss health itself.

Health is never static. There are changing levels of wellness, just as there are varying degrees of illness. Becoming
healthy is a process, a developing awareness that has no
end point, but allows us to experience health and happiness from moment to moment. Health is the integration of
body, mind, and spirit: the recognition that everything we
do, think, speak, feel, and believe has an impact on our
wellbeing.

We can be bored, depressed, tense, anxious, or generally
unhappy without suffering from physical illness. Being
healthy is more than the absence of bodily symptoms. And
being ill can have more than physical causes. Symptoms
are often an indication of unmet fundamental human
needs, such as recognition, a stimulating environment, love
from family and friends, or self-acceptance.

175

Illness can be a blessing, a signal guiding you back to the track of your deeper self. It can give you permission to do and say things you would otherwise suppress. It can allow you to take time off to reflect and chart a new course.

We develop diseases for honourable reasons. The needs that we fulfil through becoming ill are important and valid. When they are understood and accepted, we can move on to satisfy them in more creative ways.

Dis-ease and responsibility

While we might unconsciously "choose" our dis-ease to meet a psychological need, this idea should never be used to blame people for being unwell. Cancer and AIDS patients can suffer doubly as a result of the stigma people attach to these diseases.

The "what have you done to create this?" syndrome fails to recognize that, although we have individual identities, we are all interconnected: "I am you, you are me – your pain is my pain; your joy is my joy." If there are people out there in extreme suffering, they are part of our reality. It is a major evasion of responsibility to say: "I wonder what they did to create that illness?" It leads us to ignore poverty, starvation, injustice, and the destruction of the Earth.

If instead we accept individual as well as group responsibility, then we can give and allow help and healing freely where it is required. Humanity collectively suffers pain, and any on-going suffering represents something in our consciousness asking to be healed.

Healing is a process in which you can play a significant role. It may require you to change emotional and physical habits, and recognize that sometimes – however painfully – an illness can provide you with opportunities for self-examination, growth, and transformation. Truly effective healing encourages us to become more aware and able, in spite of life's frustrations, to live at ease with ourselves.

Healing comes from within. No remedy, in and of itself, can restore good health, just as no doctor is solely responsible for the cure. In fact, when a person is cured, but places the cure outside of themselves without addressing the "dis-ease" in their life, a new illness may appear, or the original one may return.

PREVENTION AND FEAR

Disease is a message, a part of life. We need to understand and learn from it. Then we can, ourselves, be more truly responsible for prevention.

Prevention is both about diminishing the known dangers that can make us vulnerable to dis-ease, and about an attitude, a state of mind, that encourages health.

The downside of Western preventive medicine is that it can produce fear and anxiety, which in turn can lead to dis-ease. Prevention in orthodox (conventional) terms tends to focus on screening – looking for warning signs such as lumps in the body and changes in cells. But this type of prevention can invite negativity. It implies that the body is unsafe and fragile, and will almost certainly break down. It also suggests an erroneous analogy between the human body and a machine. Moreover, Western medicine's diagnostic tools are limited. This was recently highlighted by the British Department of Health's change of policy on women's self-examination to detect breast cancer. As the original advice to search for localized lumps did not decrease mortality rates, guidelines have been modified from localized self-examination to an everyday awareness (mindfulness) of one's breasts.

Screening for disease involves the wishful thinking that most ills are preventable if detected early. This is an unrealistic expectation. In breast cancer, survival is determined not by early detection but by the biological nature of the tumour, and in the United States, for example, where mammography has been marketed for many years, mortality rates for breast cancer have not been reduced, and may even be rising. Similarly, mortality trends for cervical cancer in the United Kingdom have not been altered, despite the introduction of rigorous cervical screening.

Although life expectancy in the United States has increased, people's sense of wellness during the past 20

177

years has been declining, with nearly one half of the population unhappy about their health. Perhaps modern medicine, with its morbid attitude to prevention and screening, is contributing to a national hypochondria, "cancer-phobia", and a sense of poor health.

PREVENTION IS AWARENESS

Statistics that grimly warn of the incidence and mortality rates of cancer and heart disease are not good prevention. To counteract such negative conditioning, there needs to be positive programming about the human body's innate capacity to heal itself.

The body repairs itself daily, healing cuts and bruises, and restoring balance. From moment to moment we are being re-created. We create millions of new cells, and the energy and spirit that we have within affects the health of each cell.

The most effective way that you can promote your own good health is to be in touch with yourself, and to have an awareness of how your daily life affects your health and wellbeing. In addition, try to understand that health is a reflection of balance and flow, and that dis-ease is the result of an energy imbalance (see also pp. 37-45). Learn to respect your body, and understand that it has a healing potential of its own.

Prevention has three main aspects: Avoidance, Positive Action, and "Consciousness".

AVOIDANCE

This means not doing things that are obviously unhealthy. These would include heavy smoking, heavy alcohol consumption, drug use, having an unbalanced diet, overeating, and engaging in unsafe sex.

Avoidance is also about protecting and nurturing your body – guarding against the wind, cold, damp, and heat; avoiding long exposure of your skin to the sun; limiting the time spent in front of computer screens (VDUs), particularly during pregnancy; limiting X-ray exposure, including dental ones. If X-rays are unavoidable, ensure that a protective lead covering is placed over your vital organs.

Yin and yang
The yin-yang theory was originally described over 2000 years ago in China, by the Yellow Emperor Huang Ti. In his Classic of Internal Medicine *he envisaged a balance between two contrasting forces. One was thought to be dark, moist, watery, and female – this was known as yin. The other, called yang, was hot, dry, fiery, and male.*

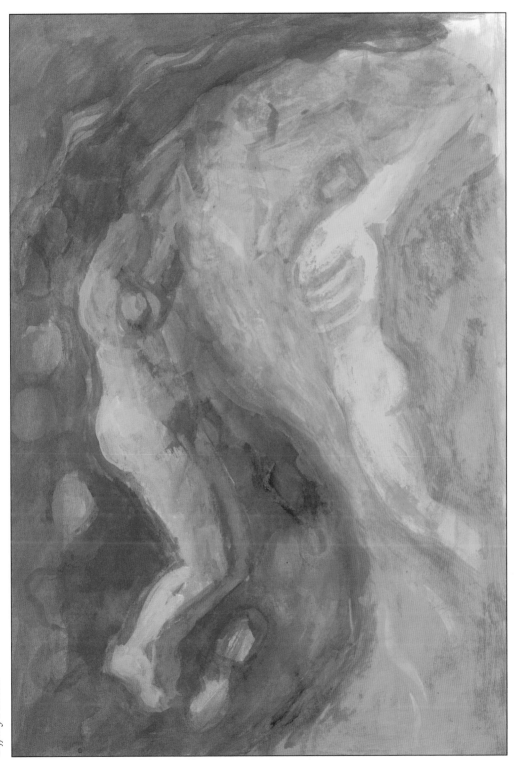

Tiffany Pearson

Care with intimate hygiene is important too. The vaginal area is chemically delicately balanced. A healthy vagina has walls lined with a protective and self-cleansing mucous membrane and a slightly acidic condition that prevents infection. It is wise to avoid using substances in or near the vagina that may upset this balance, such as tampons and bleached sanitary towels, chemically scented soaps, vaginal sprays, and douches.

POSITIVE ACTION

This is doing something healthy on a regular basis, such as eating a wholesome diet, taking exercise, and practising relaxation, yoga, and meditation, being massaged, and also developing breathing techniques, and an inner awareness.

Positive action also means developing a positive attitude toward life, and spending time nurturing and being nurtured by loved ones.

Diet

Good nutrition is essential for health. But a strict regime is not necessarily healthy, as our spiritual and mental outlook is more important than any particular diet. We should love and value ourselves, and listen to our bodies, otherwise we will not be open and motivated to follow sensible advice.

Certain foods have been found to have an adverse effect on aspects of the reproductive system. For example, according to Susan Curtis and Romy Fraser in *Natural Healing for Women* (1991), caffeine can contribute to fibroid and cyst formation; mucus-producing foods such as dairy products and red meat reduce the ability of the uterus to clean itself out during menstruation and may contribute to congestion; and alcohol can aggravate inflammatory complaints, such as cystitis. A cleansing diet may be of great benefit in conditions such as ovarian cysts, fibroids, and endometriosis.

A diet based primarily on fresh vegetables and whole-foods can reduce the input of unwanted chemicals in the body generally, and may also help prevent symptoms of congestion and inflammation developing in a woman's reproductive system.

How to become mindful of your diet

• Reduce your intake of fat by limiting red meat, avoiding fried foods, and cutting down on butter, cream, and other fatty foods

• Increase your consumption of fresh fruits, vegetables, and whole-grain cereals, which include Vitamin A, Vitamin C, Vitamin E, selenium, and dietary fibre

• Reduce your consumption of smoked and charcoal-broiled foods

• Reduce alcohol consumption

• Eliminate excess salt, refined sugar and flour, hot spices, and foods containing artificial additives or preservatives

• Reduce your consumption of coffee, tea, chocolate, and soft drinks containing caffeine

Exercise

Physical exercise benefits the body directly, through increased heart activity, and indirectly, through stimulating the immune system, which enables the mind-body to cope with stress. Physical activity, laughter, and play all produce similar positive effects on body-mind.

Relaxation, breathing awareness, and meditation

These are powerful tools: they can lower or normalize blood pressure levels, the pulse rate, and the levels of stress hormones in the blood, raise the pain threshold, and produce changes in brain-wave patterns.

Conventional medicine has only just begun to study the effects of meditation on disease, but breathing awareness is widely recognized as valuable in alleviating labour pains, and guided visualizations now form part of many alternative methods of treating cancer and other serious diseases.

Healing emotional wounds

There is growing evidence to show that negative emotions such as hopelessness, helplessness, worry, resentment, despair, grief, fear, and anger can contribute to developing dis-ease. Rather than suppressing and fighting these feelings, observe them with awareness and allow them to be. Use meditation and breathing to quieten your thoughts and emotions, and with practice, you can create an inner stillness and tranquillity. Some women may need to consult a psychotherapist or counsellor to confront and heal particularly painful or hidden trauma.

"CONSCIOUSNESS"

This involves self-awareness, to bring us more in touch with our emotions and needs. Through mindfulness we can more easily recognize and understand our ingrained patterns, and use this knowledge to keep ourselves healthy.

One way to achieve this is to become more "present", and attentive of your body, breath, thoughts, feelings, and speech. Learning how to become whole can lead to "direct experience", the experience of just being. The best way to begin is to recognize what is not your true experience – how you feel when you are out of synch and not really in your "being".

Many things interfere with how we ought to be. What we feel somebody else thinks of us, or our own judgemental thoughts of ourselves such as, "I'm useless" or, "I'm a failure", will cause interference. Observe these interferences, recognize what is not your direct experience, and let them go. When there is no interference you just are. Now and again your direct experience will emerge, and you will begin to feel it more and more.

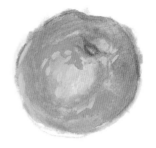

The art of mindfulness
Mindfulness is to be awake and fully aware of your body, breath, emotions, speech, and thoughts. And to be "present" with your current task, which means to stay with it, devote full attention to it, and be fully aware of it from moment to moment rather than rushing it in order to move on to the next thing. So when Zen masters say, "When eating a tangerine, eat a tangerine", they mean we need to be totally aware not just of each morsel of food in our mouth - its texture, its colour, and its flavour, but also to be present with the minute details of daily life.

Health issues

There is a unity between the different emotional and environmental situations that create dis-ease, and the time has come not to separate diseases and treatments, but rather to understand what they all have in common. Diseases do not have a life of their own. They are an individual's way of expressing ill-ease or disharmony, and are signals to lead us back on the road to a healthier life, not to be "fixed" or suppressed quickly.

The development of dis-ease is on a continuum: if a minor ailment remains untreated, it may progress to a more problematic one, and then to a more critical life issue, which may require more drastic intervention.

The disorders listed here have all been helped by competent alternative practitioners of traditional Chinese medicine, acupuncture, homeopathy, medical herbalism, and naturopathy. Other techniques that can support these main therapies include aromatherapy, shiatsu, reflexology, psychotherapy, cranial osteopathy, and osteopathy. Please note that this book is not advocating that you drop conventional treatments for the "superiority" of alternative therapies, it suggests that you combine the treatments of conventional and alternative medicine. In the event of any serious disease, it may be absolutely vital that your condition is diagnosed by a conventional doctor and equally important that you are receive treatment from an holistic practitioner.

This section is divided into five parts, but they are inter-related:

- Everyday intimate health issues
- Problematic intimate health issues
- Critical intimate health issues
- Critical life events
- Iatrogenic disorders

The treatments have not been separated from the ailments. Isolating symptoms and remedies without considering the individual cannot be holistic. While every woman is unique, the principle of combining orthodox and holistic medicine remains the same for every ailment.

For example, advice to sufferers of multiple sclerosis is to reduce consumption of animal fat and processed oils; a high intake of unsaturated fatty acids; supplement the diet with fish oils, vitamins, and minerals; avoid eating sugar and refined foods; and explore ways of reducing emotional conflict. This same advice is given for the prevention of cancer, and also for treating menstrual and menopausal distress, depression, and almost any other health problem.

The health issues are listed alphabetically. For contacts and organizations offering additional information and support see Resources, pp. 210-17.

Note: Many herbs and acupuncture points must be avoided in pregnancy. It is essential to find an experienced herbalist or acupuncurist, because indiscriminate home treatment can be harmful.

183

Contraception

Birth control is an important health issue. Deciding which method to use involves asking questions about your health, your sexual relationships, and what risks you are prepared to take. For a full discussion of contraception methods – conventional and natural and their associated risks – see pages 84-93.

If you decide to rely solely upon fertility awareness (see p. 84-9), then this will involve the willingness of your partner, to share the responsibility, and more importantly the willingness to accept pregnancy if it happens.

Menstrual and menopausal problems

Menstrual problems include pre-menstrual syndrome (PMS), the lack of periods, heavy periods, and painful periods. Menopausal distress may include hot flushes (flashes), painful lovemaking often caused by vaginal dryness, and depression.

The core of these ailments may, according to some health workers, be to do with a woman not being aware of, or feeling disconnected from, the emotional states that surround menstruation and menopause. If aspects of a woman's personality remain repressed, she can be uncomfortable with, or be in conflict with her feminine role. One extreme example is when a woman has suffered sexual abuse as a child: she may find it difficult to celebrate her sexuality and enjoy her feminine cycles and rhythms.

If you suffer from menstrual or menopausal problems, visit your doctor for a full gynaecological check-up, and take steps to improve your diet and learn how to relax more. A course of acupuncture often helps to restore hormonal balance, and meditation and yoga (see pp. 106-9, 206-7) can help reduce emotional stress.

Urinary infections

Cystitis is an infection of the urethra (urinary passage), and often *E coli* bacteria are present. Women are particularly vulnerable because the germs can be transferred from the anus to the urethra during lovemaking, on a tampon string, or through wiping the bottom from back to front.

Bruising of the vagina, sensitivity to toiletries, irritation from a contraceptive cap (diaphragm), extremes of temperature, caffeine, and spicy or acidic foods, emotional stress, and changes during the menopause can also trigger an attack.

During an attack drink plenty of fluids to flush the germs out, including soothing herbal teas such as chamomile and marshmallow. Cranberry juice is particularly effective, because it can also prevent recurrence by interfering with the bacteria's ability to stick to the bladder lining. Pau D'Arco tea, a South American herb, is excellent for cystitis and thrush.

Vaginal discharge and infections

A normal vaginal discharge is clear and slightly sticky, but if it is yellow or foul smelling there may be an infection. Known collectively as "vaginitis", vaginal infections can be caused by a forgotten tampon, chemicals in toiletries and contraceptives, a refined diet, stress, and sexually transmitted diseases.

Thrush (vaginal candidiasis) is the most common form of vaginitis, caused by an overgrowth of a normally harmless yeast (*candida albicans*), which lives in the gut. The symptoms are a white, lumpy discharge, itching, a burning sensation that is worse on passing water, and sometimes a rash. It can be triggered by the Pill, diabetes, long antibiotic courses, a poor diet, or untreated discharge.

Improve your diet by making it yeast- and sugar-free, and eat live yoghurt. Wear cotton underwear, wipe your bottom from front to back, avoid using scented toiletries, and avoid wearing tight jeans and underwear.

If, despite using natural remedies, you continue to be in extreme pain and the discharge is not clearing, conventional treatments prescribed by your doctor will provide a useful bridge during this time.

PROBLEMATIC INTIMATE HEALTH ISSUES

Benign (non-cancerous) growths

Cervical "erosion"

When cells from the inside of the cervix grow on the outside, a red, shiny area develops that may produce extra mucus, or a bloodstained discharge. The main symptom is bleeding after intercourse.

The Pill, intra-uterine contraceptive device (IUCD), trauma to the cervix, or emotional stress can all contribute to this condition. If the erosion is not painful and causes no problems it is best left alone. A course of acupuncture often helps to restore hormonal balance, and meditation and yoga can help reduce emotional stress.

Fibroids

These are non-cancerous lumps of surplus tissue in the wall of the uterus. Symptoms may include heavy, painful periods, and a swollen abdomen.

Small fibroids usually cause no problem, but larger or more numerous ones can cause heavy periods, bladder irritation, bleeding between periods, and infertility. Your doctor may suggest hormonal treatment, which prevents the ovaries from making estrogen, as fibroids are dependent on estrogen. However, this may produce menopausal symptoms. Alternatively s/he may advise surgery to remove them. If they are too large or too numerous s/he may suggest a hysterectomy, but this should always be a last resort. As with all the ailments in this section, homeopathy and acupuncture can both help.

Endometriosis

When parts of the lining of the womb attach themselves to other areas of the pelvis (the ovaries, fallopian tubes, or the outside of the uterus), they grow and bleed each cycle, just as if they were still inside the womb. The blood forms scar tissue, causing parts of the organs to stick together.

Symptoms include heavy, painful periods, pain between periods and during intercourse, backache, and infertility.

If you suspect endometriosis, your gynaecologist will perform a laparoscopy – a small incision through the navel – which enables him to look at your internal organs. Conventional treatments consist of hormones, surgery to scrape off affected areas, or hysterectomy. Homeopathy can be a good treatment for this condition.

Haemorrhoids

Haemorrhoids, or "piles", are swollen veins in the walls of the back passage or near the entrance to the anus. Symptoms are generally pain during bowel movements, bleeding, and itching. Straining to pass a hard bowel motion caused by a poor diet with little fibre, and lack of exercise, frequent use of laxatives, pregnancy, and anal sex, can all be contributing factors.

Improved diet, yoga positions such as shoulder- and headstands, and pelvic yoga exercises (see pp. 206-7), can help to alleviate symptoms without the necessity for drugs.

Herpes and genital warts

Herpes is caused by the Herpes simplex virus, which enters the body through the skin and mucous membranes of the mouth and genitals. There are two types: HSVI is usually characterized by cold sores or blisters on the lips and mouth; HSVII most often involves sores in the genital area.

An outbreak of genital herpes (HSVII) usually begins with a tingling or itching sensation of the skin in the genital area. There may also be a burning sensation, sores, and blisters in the vagina and on the cervix. You can contract herpes during vaginal, oral, or anal sex with someone who has an active infection.

Recurrent episodes can be triggered by stress, illness, menstruation, or pregnancy – whenever resistance to infection is lowered. Inadequate diet and drugs may also make you more susceptible to an attack. Herpes attacks are sometimes controlled with drugs.

Genital warts are caused by the Human papilloma virus (HPV) and spread during sexual intercourse with an infected partner. Symptoms are small, painless spots on the bottom of the vaginal opening. Laser treatment, or freezing the warts, is used to remove them from the area completely.

Studies show that women with HPV lesions on the cervix have an increased risk of developing cervical cancer.

Irritable bowel syndrome

Irritable bowel syndrome (IBS) can affect any part of the digestive tract. Common symptoms include bloating, diarrhoea/constipation, and abdominal pain. It is thought to be stress-related and may also be provoked by food intolerance, former gut infections, or candidiasis.

Eat regular, balanced meals and avoid foods that upset you. Avoid unnecessary antibiotics and drugs, and explore ways of expressing, rather than repressing, your feelings.

Osteoporosis

This is loss of bone density, and affects one in four women after menopause. Those most at risk are women who have had an early menopause, a hysterectomy and removal of the ovaries before menopause, or who eat a diet low in calcium and exercise excessively, or who smoke or drink heavily.

You can help prevent the onset of osteoporosis before menopause by eating a calcium-rich diet to build up the bones, and exercising adequately to build up strength and good bone density. Orthodox treatments are Hormone Replacement Therapy (HRT) and drugs.

Ovarian cysts

A cyst usually develops when a follicle has grown large, as happens naturally every month during ovulation, but has failed to rupture and release an egg. Most of these cysts fill with fluid; others become solid, usually benign, tumours.

Ovarian cysts are relatively common, and often do not cause any pain. Symptoms may include a disturbance in the menstrual cycle, pain or discomfort in the lower abdomen, pain during sex, and unexplained abdominal swelling. Seek advice from your doctor if you develop any of these symptoms.

Ovarian cysts are usually found during a routine bimanual pelvic examination (see pp. 201-2), and generally disappear themselves, although some may have to be removed.

To determine whether this is necessary, your gynaecologist will use ultrasound or laparoscopy (see p. 186), and a tissue sample will reveal if the cyst is benign or malignant. Doctors disagree about the necessity for removing benign cysts. In most cases, removal is unnecessary and should be avoided since ovaries perform many functions, even after the menopause. Recurrent cysts indicate an imbalance, and alternative approaches to healing could help to restore harmony to your system.

Pelvic inflammatory disease (PID)

This is an umbrella term for infections that attack the reproductive organs. Pelvic pain should never be ignored, as untreated it can cause infertility. The most common culprit is Chlamydia, a sexually transmitted disease, but other triggers can be vaginal infections following childbirth, an abortion, or the insertion of an IUCD. Symptoms range from mild and barely noticeable to acute pelvic pain, bleeding after sex or between periods, weight loss, diarrhoea, tiredness, backache, pain on passing water, and infertility. As PID is a major cause of blocked fallopian tubes – and hence infertility – it is important to diagnose and treat it quickly.

Usually the gynaecologist will prescribe a course of strong antibiotics and advise rest until the symptoms clear up. Your partner should also be investigated for an infection, and treated, to prevent recurring PID. If the symptoms persist, the gynaecologist may perform a laparoscopy (see p. 186) to rule out any other causes of pain. If you suffer from recurrent pelvic infections, become aware of your particular triggers, avoid stress, and change your lifestyle by getting extra rest and relaxation.

Prolapse

A prolapse happens when the muscles of the pelvic floor become slack and no longer support the pelvic organs adequately. In severe cases, the ligaments and tissues that hold the uterus in place may also weaken, and the uterus may "fall into" the vagina.

Symptoms are a tendency to leak urine when you cough, sneeze, or laugh suddenly, and you may have a dull, heavy sensation in your vagina, or feel as if something is falling out.

There are two main causes:

• Normal childbirth does not usually harm the ligaments, but if the labour is very rapid, or if it is a forceps delivery, this may weaken the ligaments, laying the foundations for a prolapse later on.

• The normal forces of gravity create constant downward pressure. Chances of a prolapse are higher if you have a chronic cough that creates high pressure day after day, chronic constipation, which will make you strain, and a weight problem that puts pressure on the supporting structures.

The best prevention is to increase the fibre in your diet to avoid constipation, and to do regular pelvic exercises (see p. 206) and leg lifts , which strengthen the muscles of the pelvic floor and lower abdomen. You may also strengthen a slightly prolapsed uterus by relaxing in the knee-chest position (kneeling with your chest on the floor and your bottom in the air) several times a day. Some yoga positions, such as shoulder and head stands, may relieve discomfort.

Many gynaecologists suggest a retaining vaginal ring pessary first for a prolapse, and if this is not effective hysterectomy, but this should only be considered as a last resort.

Psycho-sexual problems

Children begin life as innocent beings; their movements, energy, and expressions of love are uninhibited and flowing. Research has shown that if, during our early years, we are loved, held, admired, and respected we build up a healthy self-image. This natural vitality can gradually become constrained through the well-intentioned, but negative, conditioning of family and society. Many of us grow up believing that our natural way of being is wrong, which can cause us to suppress feelings of desire, arousal, and adventure.

We come to fear our ability to feel pleasure. When we tighten and contract to avoid pain and rejection, the energy flow stops. To be sensitive and open to love means to be vulnerable and open to hurt, so we hold back. Our energies remain locked in certain parts of the body and we build a protective armour – emotional and physical – from what we perceive as the threat of feeling deeply. This tightening can take place anywhere in the body – not just in the vaginal area – and still affect us sexually.

Women who do not experience orgasm, who suffer from lack of arousal, or who are unable to tolerate penetration (vaginismus), may be unconsciously expressing a fear of letting go and an inability to feel safe enough to experience love, sexuality, and vitality.

A sexual problem is an indication that the mind-body has been wounded. Therefore, sex therapy should aim to help the person learn to identify her wounded areas by exploring those parts that have been rejected, ignored, or denied. To heal them we need to give our wounds recognition, care, tenderness, and love.

To release and heal wounded emotions, an enlightened programme would combine counselling for both partners, with deep massage, breathing awareness, movement, and expression.

Holistic sex therapy would primarily focus on healing birth trauma, childhood emotional wounds, and current relationships. Employing the use of counselling and sensate focus techniques (massage, foreplay, caressing) can also be helpful.

Undiagnosed pelvic pain

If doctors cannot find an obvious cause, some may just dismiss pelvic pain as "psychological" – "all in the woman's head". This is where alternative therapy shines. No symptom is dismissed, every one is valid, and technology can sometimes be useful in diagnosis.

Urinary incontinence

After pregnancy, and more commonly around the time of menopause, some women begin to notice a slight loss of urine when they cough, sneeze, laugh, or exert themselves. However, incontinence in women is not an inevitable result of becoming older. It always has a cause, which may include: a bladder infection such as cystitis; constipation (which puts extra pressure on your organs), certain medications such as tranquillizers, antihistamines, and diuretics; some medical conditions such as diabetes, multiple sclerosis, or Parkinson's disease; depression, anxiety, or bereavement; pregnancy in the later months, which may weaken bladder control; difficult childbirth, which can damage the pelvic floor muscles, and obesity, which can put pressure on the pelvic floor and bladder.

Apart from surgery (see FRS, pp. 194-5), treatment for stress incontinence would include exercises to strengthen the pelvic floor muscles, and learning how to stop your urine in mid-flow. You could also visit an incontinence advisor.

CRITICAL INTIMATE HEALTH ISSUES
Abnormal smear (pap) test result

Learning that you have an abnormal smear (pap) test, and its possible connection with cervical cancer, can result in a myriad of emotions and thoughts: disbelief, fear, a sense of vulnerability, anger, and many more emotions. Every woman feels the impact in some stressful way. Smears aid in the discovery, and possi-

189

ble reversal, of a more serious disease. Smear tests detect an abnormal process that has already begun. Approximately 50% of smear results are inaccurate, however, and some abnormal smear results disappear without any obvious cause.

An abnormal smear result usually does not mean cancer. It is not a critical situation unless the smear (pap) reading reports invasive cancer, because abnormal growth takes time to occur.

The "class" system is used to name the kind of cells found in your cervix, and there are five major classifications:

Class I: Normal smear (pap), no abnormal cells

Class II: Atypical cells present, but no cancer

Class III: Abnormal cells showing mild to moderate disorganized cell growth patterns (dysplasia)

Class IV: Abnormal cells showing severe dysplasia

Class V: Invasive cancer

If your smear (pap) test is atypical or abnormal, your gynaecologist has many other tests available to determine exactly what the problem is. S/he may use a colposcope, an instrument that magnifies the surface of the vagina and cervix, to pinpoint suspicious areas for biopsy (removal of cervical tissue). Hysterectomy should be the last option.

Minor abnormalities in your cervical cells can be caused by inflammation from untreated chronic infections such as herpes, chlamydia, or thrush. Trauma to the cervix can also be caused by cervical caps (diaphragms), cervical sponges, infected intra-uterine contraceptive device (IUCD) strings, and tampons. Infections can produce cellular irregularities that mimic more serious disorders.

The cervix can be vulnerable to irritating substances, such as talc and vaginal deodorants, so avoid using them.

AIDS and sexually transmitted diseases (STDs)

AIDS and STDs are critical issues in every woman's life: any one of us can develop any of these diseases. AIDS is a collective responsibility because we are all interconnected.

More than any other condition, AIDS has dramatically altered our lives. It has made us examine our sexual habits, health care, and the doctor-patient relationship, and in all these areas it is bringing about changes in attitudes.

The most effective treatments are prevention through awareness of safer sexual practices, compassion and care for those suffering from the effects of the virus, and improved communication and consciousness throughout the planet to prevent further spread.

Facing the sun
The sun's light reflected in the face represents the possibility of new life and hope for the future. It also relates to a pregnant woman's willingness, and even willing, to nurture and create new life.

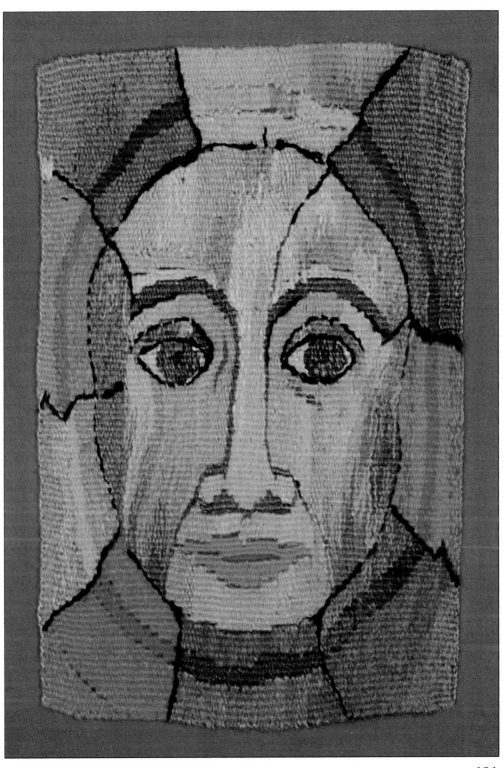

Sue Reeves

Breast disease

Many women experience tender breasts (mastalgia) during the menstrual cycle; this is thought to be a result of the body reacting to its own hormones.

Following the recent British government health report questioning the value of regular self-examination, the new guidelines advise on breast awareness on a daily basis.

Look for any changes in the outline or shape of the breast, especially those caused by arm movement, or any puckering or dimpling, lumps, thickening, or bumpy areas in one breast or armpit, and for changes in nipples. New and persistent pain should be investigated.

Mammography (breast X-ray) only remains a valid diagnostic test for a suspicious lump. Many experts question its value as a way of detecting small changes in breast tissue, especially in younger women.

Mastectomy

A mastectomy is the removal of one or both breasts, and is usually performed after invasive cancer has been detected in the area. Having a mastectomy can be a devastating emotional and physical experience.

For men: If your partner has had a mastectomy, it is essential for her to be physically intimate. The resumption of loving, not necessarily sexual, activity is crucial for a full recovery – caresses, hugs, and kisses are always possible.

For women: Your partner may need counselling, to help him adapt to changes in your body. Couples often find that surviving painful life events can reinforce an unshakeable foundation on which to build the rest of their lives.

Note: Ensure that a mastectomy is carried out during the most favourable time of your cycle (see p. 101-2).

Silicone implants and cosmetic surgery

In 1992, concern was raised in the United States regarding the possible long-term effects to women who have undergone silicone implants. This concern has brought into question the health risks of women's cosmetic surgery in general.

Cosmetic surgery is the fastest growing "medical" specialization. According to Naomi Wolf in *The Beauty Myth* (1990), more than two million Americans, 87% of them female, had undergone cosmetic surgery by 1988. Society rewards beauty on the outside over health on the inside. In the struggle for women's equality the one subject that is still taboo is women's compulsive pursuit of beauty. If a political regime subjected its people to some of the atrocities that women endure in the name of "beauty'" there would be an international outcry.

Cancer of the reproductive organs

Although the causes of cancer are not clearly understood, it is widely acknowledged that there are many interrelated factors. Genetic, environmental, dietary, and lifestyle influences can all cause and/or contribute to cancer.

Genetic factors
• Hereditary traits and tendencies may be passed on by parents in their genes. These may be not only physiological in origin, but also include emotional patterns of behaviour. Drugs can also be involved, for example, a drug called Diethylstilboestrol (DES) given to women in the 1960s to prevent miscarriage has been linked to cancer in a number of their daughters

Environmental factors
• Pollutants in the work place, such as asbestos and radiation
• Pollutants in the environment, such as lead and aluminium
• Substances such as nitrates in pickled and smoked foods,
• Substances in tampons and sanitary towels, such as dioxins
• Passive smoking
• Long-term exposure to the sun
• Unnecessary X-rays

Diet and lifestyle factors
• Heavy smoking
• Heavy alcohol consumption
• Excessive fat intake
• Consumption of hormones in meat
• Long-term use of steroids and hormones such as the Pill and hormone replacement therapy (HRT)
• Recurrent exposure to genital viruses
• On-going and unexpressed emotional stress

Cervical cancer
The symptoms are bleeding between periods, bleeding after menopause, after intercourse, after a pelvic examination or douching, and unusual, or foul-smelling vaginal discharge.

Studies report that women who douche more than twice a week may be at an increased risk of cervical cancer: douching removes normal vaginal secretions and kills healthy bacteria.

Endometrial (uterine) cancer
A malignancy of the uterine (womb) lining. The most common symptoms include bleeding or watery, bloody discharge after menopause, bleeding between periods, or increased bleeding during periods, and unusual discharge, or spotting.

Ovarian cancer
Malignancy of the ovaries. Symptoms can include a vague pressure in the pelvis or abdomen, an uneasy feeling in the stomach area, distension or bloating, enlarged abdomen, abnormal vaginal bleeding, chest problems, coughing, pressure, difficulty in breathing, and flu-like symptoms.

There are usually no symptoms or tests that can diagnose ovarian cancer. During a pelvic examination, if the gynaecologist can feel an enlarged ovary, he may use ultrasound for confirmation and a laparoscopy (see p. 186) to confirm diagnosis and subsequent treatment.

193

Hysterectomy and female reconstructive surgery (FRS)

Hysterectomy is the surgical removal of the uterus. It is the most frequently performed major surgical procedure in the United States, surpassed only by Caesarean section. Yet many hysterectomies are not necessary. They continue to be performed unnecessarily because, as part of a male-centred society, women have become culturally conditioned to accept that the loss of their reproductive organs is a real possibility after menopause, if they are suffering from uterine problems.

Traditionally, many gynaecologists consider a woman's reproductive organs as being distinct from the rest of her. But, like all our organs, they do not exist in isolation, disconnected from other systems. It is important to retain one's uterus, even after menopause, as it plays a vital role in maintaining good pelvic anatomy. The ovaries are also vital, even after menopause, as they stimulate organs, tissues, and body functions.

Female reconstructive surgery (FRS), as pioneered by American gynaecologist Vicki Hufnagel, ensures that in cases of benign (non-cancerous) disease, a woman's uterus, ovaries, and associated tissues and organs are repaired, rather than removed. It can provide an alternative to hysterectomy for millions of women, and avoids many of the usual – but commonly ignored – complications that may follow a hysterectomy, including bladder and urinary problems, prolapse, bowel complications, loss of ovarian function leading to osteoporosis, depression, loss of sexual desire, and painful intercourse.

Although FRS is a more creative example of a surgical procedure that honours the feminine body, rather than castrates it, perhaps surgery could be avoided totally if the woman had had less invasive treatments and had generally been more healthy in the first place. FRS has "married" the precision of surgical skills with the gentle, healing properties of natural substances such as amino acids and vitamins. Patients are put on a course of vitamins before surgery; and during surgery the tissues are infused with natural solutions to prevent adhesions; and post-operatively further amino acids and vitamins are administered to promote healing.

Questions to ask yourself before considering a hysterectomy
• Are you conscious of your puberty, first menstruation, and early sexual activity, and have you healed these early wounds?
• Do you understand that your menstrual cycle is a healing power source?
• Does your diet support your healing process or hinder it?
• Is your illness an unspoken communication that you need to express?
• Do you believe that you have the ability to heal yourself and can be healthy, and have you explored alternative methods of

healing?

• Do you reach out for love and support and surround yourself with people who love and support your healing process?

• What is in the way of healing yourself? That is, are you following your authentic feelings and being true to your life's purpose?

Infertility

Infertility is the inability to conceive. It is estimated that one in six couples will experience fertility problems, and in Britain alone there are some two million people whose lives are affected this way. Infertility can be devastating and humiliating for a couple. Infertility appears to be on the increase, although there are no statistics to confim this.

There can be many possible causes, such as heredity, poor diet, too much alcohol and heavy smoking, post-Pill sterility, sterility caused by intra-uterine devices (IUCDs), tight pants and hot baths (for men the testes must remain cool), sterility caused by sexually transmitted diseases, delayed child bearing due to later marriages or economic instability, and other, unexplained factors.

Steps to minimize the risk of infertility

• Improve your overall and reproductive health, which will improve your fertility

• Take care to avoid the use of invasive methods of contraception such as the Pill and the intra-uterine contraceptive device (IUCD), which can cause infections to the fallopian tubes

• Ensure that any genito-urinary infections or sexually transmitted diseases that you and your partner suffer from do not go undiagnosed and untreated

• Avoid eating junk foods

• Avoid, limit, or protect your organs from X-rays, including dental ones

• Try to find ways of healing any conflict and emotional stress in your life.

Infertility is an area where bridging the gap between conventional and complementary medicine could be very effective, as technology could be used in conjunction with natural and spiritual approaches. A woman receiving in vitro fertilization, which is intrusive to the body, could be offered homeopathy and/or acupuncture to make the procedure more balanced. Technological treatments done with love and integrity are not against Nature. It is only when technology does not embody these qualities that it becomes questionable.

Natural remedies for infertility should not be considered a substitute for a full medical investigation by an infertility specialist.

Ageing and infertility

A major anxiety for women during their 30s is that their biological time clock is ticking away. While a woman's fertility does decline after the age of 35, most age-related factors merely reduce your fertility rather than make you completely infertile. Statistically a good number of 40-year-olds will be able to get pregnant and have as good chance as a younger woman of having a healthy baby. Many obstetricians believe that a healthy pregnant woman of 38 is less at risk than an unhealthy younger woman. Every conception is an individual event, so there can be many influential factors, whether you are young or old.

The number of years is not as important as the way in which they were lived. For example, the quantity of X-rays that you have had in your life is more important than how old you are. How you take care of yourself – your nutrition, rest and exercise, and sexual behaviour – are more important than your age, and sometimes pregnancy is better delayed until your health is at its peak.

Positive imagery can help to counterbalance the fear-producing statistics. When you are pregnant, you are simultaneously creating the seeds of your future grand- and great-grand-children. Before you were born you already had your eggs, which carry eggs for the next generation, and so on. From this we can get the sense of "infinity", that fertility does not just begin at menarche and end at menopause. In one sense your eggs are "immortal", a very positive image if you are worried about getting older and moving past fertility.

Serious infections
Listerisa monocytogenes
Listeria is a bacterium found in rivers, soil, on vegetables, and in the gut of humans and animals. Exposure to listeria can lead to miscarriage, stillbirth, or severe illness in a newborn baby.

If you are pregnant, take practical steps to prevent listeria by avoiding soft ripened cheeses, unpasteurized dairy foods, ready-to-eat poultry, and ready prepared chilled salads. Keep raw and cooked foods apart, storing cooked on the shelf above raw in the refrigerator, and ensure that all cooked food is heated thoroughly until it is "piping hot".

Note: It may also be unwise for pregnant women, young children, and elderly people to eat raw eggs in fresh mayonnaise, meringues, and some ice cream, due to the possible presence of bacteria. However, if your level of health is fairly good then you are less susceptible.

Toxic shock syndrome
Tampon-related toxic shock syndrome (TSS) is a rare illness caused by a toxin produced by a strain of the bacteria *Staphylococcus aureus*, that is found naturally in the vagina of many women. Tampon-use can create a biological environment that encourages production of the toxin, which can cause vaginal dryness, vaginal ulcers, inflammation, and rapid loss of blood pressure, leading to respiratory and kidney failure and, in extreme cases, death.

Early symptoms are flu-like and include a high temperature, vomiting, diarrhoea, sore throat, stiff neck, headache, aching muscles, fainting and dizziness, and sunburn-like peeling rash, especially on the hands and feet or on the body. The acute phase progresses with a rapid loss of blood pressure to respiratory and kidney failure. The only way to completely eliminate the risks of TSS is to avoid using tampons altogether, but as tampons are so convenient consider the following:

Steps to minimize the risk of TSS

• Avoid high absorbency tampons. Use the lowest absorbency and change them regularly. The longer a tampon is kept in, the higher the risk

• Alternate tampons and sanitary towels and use a sanitary towel overnight

• If you have any symptoms of TSS, remove your tampon and consult your doctor immediately

Toxoplasmosis

Toxoplasmosis is an organism that can cause miscarriage, still-birth, or severe mental and physical harm to newborn babies. Toxoplasmosis is a microscopic parasite picked up from cat faeces, under-cooked and raw meat, and continental sausages. The risk arises when a woman has the infection during, or just before, pregnancy.

In France, Austria, and Spain tests for toxoplasma are routine, and if a pregnant woman is found to be infected, or has recently been infected, she is treated with antibiotics to stop the parasite crossing the placenta.

If you are pregnant, or are trying for a baby, avoid all contact with the virus. Take care not to eat undercooked or raw meats (store raw meat on the shelf below cooked food), or to handle cat-litter trays without wearing protective gloves.

CRITICAL LIFE EVENTS
Abortion (termination of pregnancy)

One of our most fundamental rights as women is to choose whether, and when, to have children. While conscious conception (see pp. 84-9) should ideally be the first defence against an unwanted pregnancy, no method is one-hundred-per-cent effective and women the world over resort to abortion when they get pregnant accidentally.

Since the introduction of pre-natal screening offered to women over the age of 35, increasing numbers of these older pregnant women are being faced with the decision of whether or not to terminate a pregnancy, if the foetus is found to be abnormal.

Whatever the circumstances surrounding a termination, few women and their partners remain untouched, and it is usually one of the most painful decisions a woman ever has to make.

If we are given an opportunity to work through our feelings beforehand, we are less likely to feel seriously depressed after the procedure. Post-abortion support groups have been set up in some areas to give women the opportunity to air their feelings, and thereby reduce emotional stress. If denied and unresolved, grief can undermine a woman's emotional wellbeing by remaining in her psyche for many years, even all her life.

Emotional trauma

Life events such as a break-up in a partnership, the death of a child or a spouse, sexual abuse as a child, or rape, can all lead to depression and illness if they remain hidden and unacknowledged. Working through these issues in order to come to terms with, and heal, a trauma may sometimes require counselling or psychotherapy.

Many "alternative" therapies work on the emotional, mental, and spiritual levels and can be very helpful and supportive during times of trauma and emotional stress.

According to Marie Beresford, a therapist and Buddhist, psycho-spiritual therapy looks at the personal and spiritual dimensions of going through the "journey of the soul". Crises are not seen as illnesses but as a time with potential for transformation, learning, and growth. Plumbing the depths of the past to heal childhood traumas is a goal shared by most forms of psychotherapy. But just as these past, and often unconscious, experiences impinge on and affect our current thoughts, and behaviour, so too there is a realm of our psyches that contain our deepest potential, the source of the unfolding pattern of our unique human path of development. It is the discovery and expression of this rich inner resource that distinguishes psycho-spiritual therapy from other forms of psychotherapy.

Miscarriage and stillbirth

Whether the miscarriage occurs in the twelfth or in the twenty-fourth week of pregnancy or whether it is full term, parents still feel the loss of a baby deeply, and their grief can be exacerbated when that fact is not recognized by society or by the health professionals caring for them. Grief that is not acknowledged and worked through can have devastating effects on the body-mind for years afterward, even a whole lifetime.

A recent British report recommends that babies miscarried after 28 weeks, and full-term stillbirths, should be given a dignified burial or cremation, and calls for changes in the way hospitals deal with such deaths, such as special training for staff involved with the parents.

Dr Peter Barr, an Australian paediatrician, who has personal experience of stillbirth in his family, encourages bereaved parents to spend time with their baby, to name it, and to take photographs, which provides them with a focus for their feelings of despair. Barr's tenderness and compassion, and his ability to address spiritual as well as medical issues, allows the bereaved parents to express their feelings, which can leave the family freer to integrate the loss of their baby and begin to come to terms with it.

Psychological distress

Women's psychological distress may be bound up with society's pressures on them to conform, to keep silent, and to fit into stereotypical roles. If women feel that they have no means of exercising choice or control over their lives, then they often resort to using their own bodies as a vehicle for their distress. This partly explains why so many psychosomatic problems such as eating disorders, and many forms of depression, affect women far more than men.

All psychological distress – be it anorexia nervosa, bulimia, or post-natal depression – needs to be addressed holistically, sympathetically, and with love and compassion. Each woman and her psychological distress is unique and individual, and treatment must be aimed at the woman not the disorder.

Post-natal depression is often treated as an illness, but perhaps it comes from a woman not having felt connected to the baby during the birth or perhaps from the very beginning of pregnancy. If a woman has not been supported during pregnancy and labour, then the whole process can become distressing rather than a celebration. A woman can help to prevent post-natal depression by becoming more mindful of her feelings and her body before, during, and after pregnancy. This can be facilitated through yoga and breathing awareness.

IATROGENIC (DOCTOR- AND DRUG-INDUCED DISORDERS)
'Iatrogenic' is a term used to describe an illness or condition produced in a patient by the actions of a physician or of a medical treatment. With particular regard to women's intimate health care, iatrogenic illness most commonly hap-

pens in obstetric units and family planning clinics. In obstetric units unnecessary episiotemies and caesareans can create lasting problems. In family planning clinics , some women who have been subjected to particularly painful pelvic examinations have developed vaginismus as a result. Women have been found to suffer bladder infections from cap (diaphragm) usage, ovarian cysts from intra-uterine devices (IUCDs), and vaginal infections from over-prescribed antibiotics.

However, iatrogenic illness does not only involve doctors and treatments – it can include everyday feminine products such as "hygiene" sprays, tampons and sanitary towels that contain harmful ingredients such as dioxins.

Mass drugging and mass vaccination without real knowledge of the long-term effects of either might play a larger role than we currently realize in the onset of even more serious diseases. Very often the main part of any holistic treatment is helping the patient to reduce or make only necessary use of medication, and follow advice on an improved diet and lifestyle.

Pelvic health and examinations
Western diagnostic medicine has tended to focus on examining a particular organ in isolation from the rest of the person. Physical examinations are not the only way to gain knowledge and prevent disease; noticing changes in our menstrual

cycle, loss of appetite, or any unusual pain should all form part of prevention.

The value of pelvic and self-examinations should not be dismissed, and you should always visit your gynaecologist for diagnosis of any problem. However, without mindfulness (see p. 28), such pelvic examinations cannot be considered holistic. Body awareness, together with a pelvic examination, would be the ideal combination.

THE PELVIC EXAMINATION

Part of every Western woman's health checks throughout her life will almost certainly be regular pelvic examinations. The experience can vary from woman to woman: one may tolerate it without any difficulty, another may be totally unable to relax and allow the doctor to examine her.

Most of us tend to fall between these two extremes, but much depends on the attitude and behaviour of the examining physician. Some women prefer a female doctor to examine them vaginally, while others have no preference. The doctor's gender need not be a crucial factor so much as his or her quality of care.

The origins of many physical illnesses may be emotional, and the symptoms may be manifest in women's reproductive organs. For example, conditions such as vaginismus – the inability to allow intercourse – may reveal themselves during a pelvic examination. To treat a bodily symptom that has an emotional basis, a gynaecologist should be prepared to address a woman's spiritual, psychological, and emotional needs.

It can help immensely during a vaginal examination if the gynaecologist is able to honour and respect the soul of the patient. She or he should be someone who is respectful of the being of the patient, of the fact that the woman s/he is examining has a world of experience and feelings happening at that moment; someone who is not removing herself mentally from the examining room.

A spiritual gynaecologist would have a reverence for life, and for each woman's body as a manifestation of life. Such reverence would manifest itself in the doctor being in touch with her/his feminine side, by gently talking the woman through the procedure, ". . .and now I am doing this, and now I am inserting the speculum, and now I am examining this area of your body, and how is this feeling? . . ."

She or he would be constantly mindful during any pelvic examination and gynaecological procedure. S/he would possess an inner awareness of the fact that s/he is doing this procedure for a particular reason, purely for the woman's sake, and not to benefit a clinical trial. Handled insensitively, an examination, particularly in front of a crowd of medical students, can be a deeply humiliating experience.

WHAT TO EXPECT DURING AN INTERNAL EXAMINATION

Most of the fears surrounding the internal examination involve the speculum, the instrument used to open the folds of the vaginal skin to give a clear view inside. The insertion should not be painful, though it often feels uncomfortable, and if the speculum is metal, it should first be warmed.

• The gynaecologist should place a finger on the lower part of your vagina before inserting the speculum. The finger should be pressed gently down so the speculum, inserted sideways, can slide into you on the top of his finger, which prevents the speculum from scratching any part of your vagina

• The speculum should be moved slowly into the depth of the vagina, then turned to the right position and opened slowly

• Once the speculum has been inserted, the doctor will check the wall of the vagina to see if its colour is pink and healthy

• S/he will next inspect the cervix and the area around it

• At this point your doctor may take a cervical smear (Pap), which consists of swabbing cells shed from the vaginal pool and the cervix and examining them for any abnormalities (see pp. 204-5)

• Following examination of your cervix the doctor will withdraw the speculum, by turning it on its side, and slowly remove it from your vagina to avoid any pinching of the vaginal wall

• Next the doctor will conduct what is called a "bimanual" pelvic examination This begins when the doctor slides one or two fingers into your vagina, and with them inside puts his finger on your cervix and gently moves it. S/he will then place her/his other hand on your abdomen

• As s/he gently presses on your abdomen, s/he will slowly tilt your uterus by pushing the cervix from the inside, which helps to determine the position and size of your uterus. (The position of your womb does not make any difference to your health, or to your ability to have children.)

• S/he will feel your uterus for any fibroids, and also feel around the area of the fallopian tubes and ovaries. If there is any tenderness, enlargement or pain, this may indicate an infection, a growth, or endometriosis (see pp. 185-6), and the doctor may wish to perform further exploratory tests

Many women may find it immensely reassuring to be talked through the whole procedure, and even to be offered a mirror to look inside the vagina and see their cervix. Some doctors even invite the patient to hold the speculum while it is inserted, and this may be very helpful in allowing the woman to gain control over what is happening to her, and avoid discomfort.

SOME ADVICE ABOUT THE EXAMINATION
If you know vaginal examinations are a problem for you, tell the doctor who is to

examine you, and enlist his/her co-operation and compassion.

When you are asked to lie down on the examination table with your knees apart, you will find that your whole pelvic area relaxes if you can allow your waist and bottom to sink heavily on to the table. Deep relaxed breathing will also help.

Try to explore with the gynaecologist the positions in which you feel most comfortable being examined, as different positions can help many women during internal examinations. Cultural bias rather than scientific fact often determines certain practices. In some countries internals are done with the woman lying on her side.

If your gynaecologist is enlightened, s/he may be able to suggest alternative examining positions that can help to release the muscles of the pelvic floor. These positions derive from yoga postures and are used to reduce the pain of labour, and ease delivery by going with the force of gravity. They are instinctive – natural yet forgotten – movements that can be practised daily to help relax and open the pelvis. While these new positions may feel strange at first, they are certainly worth a try, especially if traditional methods do not succeed.

Positions to relax the pelvis

• In the first position, squat on the floor with your feet apart, flat on the floor, and your hands holding the back of a chair for support. The gynaecologist can introduce examining fingers from the side or front. This position can also help reduce the pain of menstrual cramps (see p. 184)

• Another position is a variation on the first: you squat on the floor and lean forward on to a chair or cushions. The examination can be carried out from behind

The most important factor that can enable a nervous woman to undergo pelvic examinations is an unconscious one: the gynaecologist's ability to tolerate or hold her/his patient's fear.

During an examination it is common for a frightened woman to want to push feelings of pain, fear, and disgust on to the gynaecologist, in the hope that she can get back something that will take away those emotions and replace them with good feelings. This is "projection" (see pp. 61-2), whereby we unconsciously put unwanted parts of ourselves into others. During infancy it is one's mother who normally acts as the "container" for some of these intolerable fears and feelings. In a sense, the gynaecologist needs to become a good container during the examination by not retaliating, that is, by not becoming angry if you tense up and prevent him/her from examining you.

If the doctor is able to bear your fear, as well as tolerate the impotence it makes her/him feel if s/he cannot complete an examination, then your fears can be turned into good feelings. You will be able to tolerate the examination because the doctor can hold the pain and anxiety that an examination may arouse.

Unfortunately, these issues may not be addressed in general medical training, and many doctors may not think of the woman's feelings – conscious or unconscious – as they examine her.

A NOTE TO EXAMINING PHYSICIANS

It is perhaps less well known or obvious that a positive, sensitive pelvic examination can have therapeutic value for the woman who suffers from vaginismus. My personal experience confirms that a gentle pelvic examination can be a positive step toward reversal of both vaginismus, and the fear of being vaginally examined.The gynaecologist may be the first person a vaginismus sufferer approaches. If she receives no help from her/him, she may feel unable ever again to ask for help from anyone else. Similarly, if a woman has an extreme fear of pelvic examinations, and she is not treated sympathetically, she may avoid further gynaecological check-ups, including vital cervical smears (Pap tests).

The advantage of treating vaginismus at the primary care level is that it can be dealt with when it first appears, before it becomes reinforced. Vaginismus may first appear in a young woman asking for contraception. If you have difficulties in giving her a cervical smear (Pap) test, you should be able to recognize her condition as possible vaginismus and explore it with her. Since early diagnosis and help can prevent a woman from seeking inappropriate treatment, I believe it is vital for as many gynaecologists as possible to receive training in treating vaginismus.

The nature of vaginismus makes it a particularly sensitive and delicate issue, therefore it is important that greater focus be placed on gentleness and awareness during the pelvic examination. Vaginismus challenges many unconscious fears and may produce internal conflicts in the doctor confronted with it. It might make you feel powerless because it prevents you from being able to examine a woman, but through increased awareness you can be helped to understand that she is not consciously resisting examination.

WAYS TO IMPROVE THE PELVIC EXAMINATION FOR ANXIOUS WOMEN

• During their first consultations with you, many women suffering from vaginismus will be unable to do more than talk and allow you to touch the entrance to the vagina with the tip of your finger
• Your response to a woman's fear should be firm but reassuring, without rejecting her (in extreme cases she may shake and express the urge to vomit, or move away from you toward the top of the examination table)
• Encourage the woman to "go into" her fear instead of turning away, and reassure her that although you regret the degree of her trauma, it is safe for her to shake and even to vomit
• Suggest that she places her hands on the insides of her thighs

203

to try to keep her legs from trembling, then hold a mirror in front of her vulva, and help her to sit up slightly so that she can see

• Point out the opening of her vagina, and slowly encourage her to touch her vagina and gently insert a finger

• You will need to reassure the woman that speedy progress need not be a priority, since everyone goes at their own pace. However, at times it may be appropriate to point out that her need to remain passive and go slowly forces you to push things along. Ask her how this makes her feel. Encouraging the woman to recognize that she is no longer a vulnerable person can help her to see how she can risk being less passive, so that she can become more powerful and ultimately more responsible

• The most important factor that can enable terrified women to undergo a full pelvic examination or gynaecological procedures will be your ability to tolerate her fear and panic. You need to be able to "contain" these feelings during the examinations, and you can do this by not retaliating. "Not retaliating" means that you do not try to suppress, make light of, or become angry at the woman's suffering and fear. You are able to bear her panic, as well as tolerate the impotence she might make you feel whenever the muscle spasm is too strong for you to complete an examination

• Finally, at the end of every consultation, you and your patient should discuss her feelings during the examination. You can convey to her that you are not completely invulnerable, but are able to cope and accept her anxieties. Through these consistent exchanges the woman can discover that she has enough strength within her and is resilient enough to bear panic and fear without feeling destroyed

• The fear of being examined can be understood and worked through, simply because you are able to give these feelings your deepest attention during the examinations, and be there for her, in the same way that a good parent is for her/his child

THE CERVICAL SMEAR (PAP) TEST

The cervical smear (Pap) test – was developed by Dr George Papanicolaou over 50 years ago, and is used to diagnose cancer of the cervix and other infections.

The cervix is known to be a delicate and vulnerable area, where women have the potential to become seriously ill. If we could be assured that smear (Pap) test results were accurate, women might feel more confident about them. Perhaps we need to ask why the cervix is such a vulnerable area to cancer. It is best to have this awareness, so that it can be prevented in certain vulnerable women, even though too much focus on it can produce unnecessary fear.

The most common way for a gynaecologist to take a smear (Pap) test is to examine your whole cervix through a speculum, then, using a wooden spatula, s/he will take a full circular scrape of the area. When the doctor takes your smear, ask to see your cervix. S/he probably has a mirror handy, and perhaps s/he can point out particular areas or any inflammation to you.

PREPARING FOR A SMEAR (PAP) TEST

• The smear should be done before a bimanual (see p. 201) examination is performed, that is, when the gynaecologist feels your cervix, uterus, and ovaries with one hand on your abdomen, and two fingers inside your vagina
• The best time to take a smear (Pap) test is just before or at ovulation (see pp. 81-2), when the estrogen level is high. The cells are flatter and easier for the laboratory technician to read. Knowledge of your own cycle is important to achieve a more accurate result (see pp. 80-4)
• It is inadvisable to have a smear test during menstruation and for a few days after, because blood interferes with the reading of the cells
• After an intra-uterine contraceptive device (IUCD) is removed, smears should not be taken until at least one month has

elapsed. IUCDs, due to inflammation caused by strings hanging down through the cervical opening into the vagina, can cause cells to mimic abnormal cancerous cells
• Swimming, bathing, and sexual intercourse have not been found to affect a smear (Pap) test. Douching will disturb the cervical cells and the use of medications, herbal remedies, and spermicides may affect the slide. The fewer chemical and other matters immediately in your vaginal area, the more accurate the sample will be
• Drugs that may affect smear (Pap) test results are antibiotics, cancer therapy drugs, allergy injections, thyroid drugs, antihistamines, valium, and aspirin. Steroids for asthma or arthritis have also been found to hinder the ability of the body to fight abnormal cell growth
• After any procedure that disturbs the cells on the cervix, it is unwise to repeat the smear before a new layer of cells has reached the surface, otherwise a false reading may result. Wait a minimum of one to three months before repeating the test

Yoga relaxation can ease pelvic examinations, cervical smears (Pap) tests, or other gynaecological procedures

While you can focus some yoga postures on the pelvic area, the main thing always is the breathing. To reduce anxiety and muscle spasm during a pelvic examination or gynaecological procedure, the breathing technique has to be very strong and confident, something that you can become very good at. Practise the following exercises at home before an examination so that you will be able to apply some, if not all, of them when you need them the most.

PELVIC YOGA EXERCISES

• Start the routine by lying on your back. Bend your knees, put your feet parallel on the floor so that they are grounded, with your feet slightly wider apart than the width of your hips. Give yourself a big hug to open the space between the shoulder blades, and let your arms move away to make space for the spine

• Close your eyes, tune in to your breath without changing it, and stay with the breath for a while. Observe your mind, and how it wanders. Recognize your thoughts, otherwise they are affecting you without your being aware of them. Acknowledge that they are there, and by acknowledging them, the conflict almost dissolves

• Continue watching your breath until it becomes more rhythmical. Feel the gravity, let your back sink to the floor. The more you surrender to gravity, the freer the whole body becomes. Your pelvis is the biggest bone in your body, and the base of the spine is the thickest and heaviest part of the spine. By putting the emphasis on the exhalation to empty your lungs and release the upper body, you will allow your pelvis to sink deep, deep, down to the ground

• The back of your pelvis is sinking. Now get in touch with the symmetry: feel whether the right and left sides of your pelvis are evenly on the floor, feel the backbone (sacrum) and become familiar with it. Get in touch with the ground so that it becomes your security. Continue breathing and observing thoughts that come up to block the breath

• It takes a lot of practice just to allow your back to sink to the floor, and in that sinking your internal organs, your vagina, and everything else inside you, can open like a flower, because you have a stem, a root

• Yoga is about getting in touch with that security, in order to allow that opening to come. If you have no connection to the ground, then naturally it is very frightening to open, because like a flower, you fear you're going to be picked. But if you've got a deep root and you keep planting the root, you're not going to be picked. A flower could, but you are actually deep in your being, in your roots. Whatever is happening, is happening on the surface

• Go into that place and stay deep within yourself, and you will realize that the doctor is not touching you there. What is being touched is the exterior, but not your core, not your heart. You do not feel the need to tense up because you are deep, deep in your core where you are so grounded that you can allow your periphery to be examined, and even deep inside your vagina is still not you. You are deeper than that, because where you are is the invisible centre

• If you are doing all this and then suddenly you feel panic and your vagina tightens, it might be very difficult to do anything further at this stage. Try breathing and letting go, and ask the doctor to stop until you feel ready again. However, if you have practised this way of mindfulness often enough and have become familiar with thoughts that come up, then when they arise during the examination they won't have the same power. They are familiar to you. If the panic comes up, this practice can help you to learn how to do nothing, to learn how to say, "I am feeling panic as the speculum is entering me, and I am breathing in", and "I am experiencing discomfort as the smear is being taken, and I am breathing out"

• Slowly, instead of the panic taking you over, you are inviting it in and joining it up with your breath, so that you are still breathing. Panic is something that comes on through thought and when we panic we cannot breathe. If you can continue to breathe in and out, the panic will dissolve because you are breathing rhythmically

• Become good at practising this alone. Then, when the gynaecologist wants to examine you, you have a skill – a feminine secret – whereby you know how to allow yourself to open without losing yourself, because you have a deep, secure ground of your being

SELF-EXAMINATION

Many women feel that examining their vagina is an important part of the process of taking control of, and responsibility for, their own bodies. Looking at the cervix regularly with the help of a speculum to open the vaginal walls, can help you recognize your fertile days, pregnancy, and spot early signs of infection or cellular changes that might indicate more serious problems. The cervix changes throughout the month with your cycle and if you check it regularly you may be able to notice changes.

One way to learn about self-examination is as part of a women's health group, where the support of others can help with the initial difficulties of using a speculum (the metal or plastic instrument used by doctors to open the vagina for examination). A group also offers the unique opportunity to see other women's genitals, which can give you a reassuring sense of the range of shapes that vaginas and cervixes can be.

How to conduct a self-examination

You will need a mirror, a torch, a speculum, and a natural oil such as almond oil. Before you insert the speculum, practise opening and closing it.

• Settle yourself comfortably, lean against something such as a bed and relax your stomach muscles

• Insert a finger inside your vagina to feel where your cervix is, so that you know the direction to point the speculum in

• Point your finger at the top of the crease of your bottom

• Put some oil on the speculum, and spread your labia open with one hand

• Point the speculum at the small of your back and slide it in gently. Some women find it easier to slide it in on its side. After it is past the strong ring of muscles at the opening of your vagina, it should go in fairly easily

• Once the speculum seems to have gone in far enough (for some women this is half of its length, for others the whole of it), open it up slowly a couple of notches

• Have a look with the help of a torch and a mirror. Your vaginal walls will usually be pale pink and very crinkly, and you should be able to see your cervix in the end of the speculum. Coughing sometimes brings it into view!

• Your cervix is smooth and round, and you will be able to see the hole in the middle (the os), which is the opening into your uterus

• A healthy cervix is shiny, smooth, and even, varying in colour from pale pink to red, acquiring a bluish tinge in pregnancy and just before a period in some women. At ovulation, around two weeks before your next period, the os opens and the secretion from it changes from being white, sticky, and slight, to a clear, slippery, thin mucous

• The cervix, like your skin, can be an indicator of your general state of health

• Get to know the smell and texture of your normal vaginal secretions so that you can spot any changes. A peculiar-smelling, or odd-coloured discharge is often an early sign of infection. Accepting your own menstrual blood, vaginal smell, taste, and secretions is part of owning your vagina, and learning to love your body and your inner self

Conclusion

As we cross the threshold into a new millennium, we are entering a critical passage of time and change. Nuclear war is no longer considered an inevitability, and the ideological and physical boundaries of past regimes, such as communism in Eastern Europe, and the Berlin Wall, have collapsed. This signals both a shift in the behaviour of the major world powers and in consciousness in general, and the integration of a feminine and spiritual dimension into medicine will also be a major element in this transition.

When we value the feeling and spiritual aspects in ourselves, we become part of an emerging spirituality, a feminine voice which speaks of:

• The recognition of the interconnectedness of all life

• The recognition of women and men as sacred and spiritual beings, and the need to love our psyches, bodies, and emotions

Restoring balance and flow to women's health care will automatically bridge the gap between orthodox, (conventional) and alternative medicine, because when a doctor harmonizes her/his feeling and intellectual sides s/he will naturally begin to integrate the two models of orthodox, (conventional) and holistic medicine into her/his approach.

But it is not just doctors who need to harmonize with these inner aspects. It is vital that we all do, because a person who chooses to become more conscious – and thereby more healthy – will inevitably create a healthier world. A healthy person would not want to live in an environment that is cruel, polluted, materialistic, and stressful, as they would not be able to live with that split in themselves. As we become whole, so too will the planet become healthier. A major part of restoring wholeness will need to include healing the relationships between women and men, since the root cause of gynaecological distress may originate from the rage and anger women feel about the abuse they have suffered from men.

But this book, has not been about championing women's causes. Although I have focused on the need to restore spiritual and feminine values to health care, current medical practice – whether carried out by male or female doctors – can injure and oppress men as much as it does women.

Feminine and spiritual principles should apply equally to medicine in general, in order to heal the female-male split, and I hope that the principles explored in this book can be used as a model for all health practices.

Health resources

There is a limit to how extensive listings such as these can be because addresses change, groups stop, and others start, etc. Use the following as a base to make your first contacts. If the listings do not include practitioners in your area, see *The Directory of Complementary and Alternative Practitioners*, available from In Position Media Group Ltd, 813 South Street, Glasgow G14 OAH Tel. (041-959 9755) or *The Holistic Network Directory*, available from The Holistic Network, PO Box 1447, London N6 5JN. Tel (081) 341 6789.

ORGANIZATIONS THAT OFFER OR CAN REFER YOU TO HOLISTIC GYNAECOLOGICAL THERAPISTS:

Association of General Practitioners of Natural Medicine, 38 Nigel House, Portpool Lane, London EC1N 7UR. Tel (071) 405-2781. *A charity for information only*

British Chiropractic Association, Premier House, 10 Greycoat Place, London SW1P 1SB. Tel (071) 222-8866.

British and European Osteopathic Association, 6 Adelaide Road, Teddington, Middx TW11 OAY. Tel (081) 977-8532.

British Holistic Medical Association, 179 Gloucester Place, London NW1 6DX. Tel (071) 262-5299. *Only GPs may contact this association for listings*

British Medical Acupuncture Society, Newton House, Newton Lane, Lower Whitley, Warrington, Cheshire WA4 41A. Tel (0925)-730727.

British Naturopathic Association, 6 Netherhall Gardens, London NW3. Tel (071) 435-7830.

The Council for Acupuncture, Suite One, 19 Cavendish Square, London W1M 9AD. Tel (071) 409-1440.

Doctor-Healer Network, Flat 2, 8 Bracknell Gardens, London NW3 7EB. Tel (071) 794-8595. (Contact: Dr Daniel J Benor MD) *A forum for health professionals to share information on integrating healing with conventional medicines*

The General Council & Register of Consultant Herbalists, Marlborough House, Swanpool, Falmouth, Cornwall TR11 4HW. Tel (0326)-317321.

General Council and Register of Osteopaths. Tel (071) 839-2060.

Holistic Aroma-Therapy, 108b Haverstock Hill, London NW3 2BD. Tel (071) 284-1315.

Incorporated Society of Registered Naturopaths, 1 Albemarle Road, The Mount, York YO2 1EN.

Institute for Complementary Medicine, PO Box 194, London SE16 1QZ. Tel (071) 237-5165.

Institute of Pure Chiropractic, PO Box 127, Oxford OX1 1HH. Tel (0865)-246687.

International Federation of Aromatherapists, Royal Masonic Hospital, Ravenscourt Park, London W6 OTN. Tel (081) 846-8066.

International Federation of Practitioners of Natural Therapeutics Ltd, 46 Pulens Crescent, Sheet, Petersfield, Hants GU13 4DH. Tel (0730)-66790.

International Institute of Reflexology, 28 Hollyfield Avenue, London N11 3BY. Tel (081) 368-0865.

International Register of Oriental Medicine, Green Hedges House, Green Hedges Avenue, East Grinstead, Sussex RH19 1DZ. Tel (0342)-313106/7.

International Society of Professional Aromatherapists (ISPA), 41 Leicester Road, Hinckley, Leicestershire LE10 1LW. Tel (0455)-637987.

National Institute of Medical Herbalists Ltd, 9 Palace Gate, Exeter EX1 1JA. Tel (0392)-426022.

Register of Traditional Chinese Medicine, 19 Trinity Road, London N2 8JJ. Tel (081) 883-8431.

Shiatsu Society, C/o 14 Oakdene Road, Redhill, Surrey RH1 6BT. Tel (0737)-767896.

Society of Homeopaths, Suite 2, 2 Artizan Road, Northampton NN1 4HU. Tel (0604)-21400.

The Tibet Foundation, 43 New Oxford Street, London WC1A 1BH. Tel (071) 379-0634. (Contact: Mr P Wangyal). *Provides referrals to Tibetan doctors*

Glasgow Homeopathic Hospital, 1000 Great Western Road, Glasgow G2. Tel (041) 339-0382.

Women Unlimited, 4A Downfield Place, Edinburgh EH11 2EW. Tel (031) 337-5543. *Offers support groups, health days, and information*

Women's Support Project, 871 Springfield Road, Glasgow G31 4HZ. Tel (041) 556-7516 & (041) 556-5205. *Offers information and resources on women's health issues*

Irish Society of Homoeopaths, Caherawoneen, Kinvara, Co. Galway. Tel (091) 3738.

Women's Clinic, British College of Acupuncture, 8 Hunter Street, London WC1N 1BN. Tel (071) 837-6429. (Contact: Dr Eunice Low and Dr Yizhen Jia)

Lotus Healing Centre, 129 Queens Crescent, London NW5 4HE. Tel (071) 284-4614 & (071) 267-4561. (Contact: Mr Gurudharam Singh Khalsa) *Chinese herbal medicine, acupuncture, yoga, and meditation*

Homeopathic Health Clinic, 29 Streatfield Road, Kenton, Middx HA3 9BP. Tel (081) 907-4885. (Contact: Dr Mrs T.A. Chhana, consulting physician in homeopathic medicine)

Holistic & Spiritual Counselling and Healing, 202 Mina Road, St. Werburghs, Bristol, Avon BS2 9YP. Tel (0272)-425727. (Contact: Elaine Heller, ITEC & Ann Coleman, SRN, ITEC, IFA)

Intuitive massage and fine energy balancing, meditation, relaxation, and self-development classes

The Natural Health Clinic, 149 Elgar Avenue, Surbiton, Surrey KT5 9JX. Tel (081) 399-9022. (Contact: Dr Donald Upton)

The Bournemouth Centre of Complementary Medicine, 26 Sea Road, Boscombe, Bournemouth, Dorset BH5 1DF. Tel (0202)-396354. (Contact: Dr Siewart, MD)

The Surgery, 20 Drury Road, Colchester, Essex CO2 7UX. (Dr Richard Laing, homeopathic medical practitioner)

The Witney Complementary Health Care Centre, 2 The Tchury, High Street, Witney, Oxon. Tel (0993)-771624. (Contact: Ann Hamilton)

Bretforton Hall Clinic, Bretforton, Vale of Evesham, Worcestershire WR11 5JH. Tel (0386)-850537. (Contact: Dr Peter Manners)

The Centre for the Study of Complementary Medicine, 51 Bedford Place, Southampton, Hants SO1 2DG. Tel (0703)-334752. *and* 6 Upper Harley Street, London NW1 4PS . Tel (071) 935-7848.

The Complementary Therapy Centre, Arndale House, St. George's Esplanade, St. Peter Port, Guernsey, Channel Islands. Tel (0481)-720708. (Contact: Drs J.N Kenyon and George Lewith)

Clissold Park Natural Health Centre, 154 Church Street, London N16 OJU. Tel (071) 249-2990 *and*: 56 Brighton Road, London N16 8EG. Tel (071) 254-5906. (Contact: Mr A. Chevallier)

Neal's Yard Therapy Rooms, 2 Neal's Yard, Covent Garden, London WC2H 9DP. Tel (071) 379-7662. (Contact: Margot McCarthy)

Acupuncture Foundation & Teaching Clinic, City Health Centre, 36 Featherstone Street, London EC1Y 8QX. Tel (071) 490-0721.

BodyWise Natural Health Centre (affiliated to the London Buddhist Centre), 119 Roman Road, London E2 OQN. Tel (081) 981-6938.

Bristol Cancer Help Centre, Grove House, Cornwallis Grove, Clifton, Bristol BS8 4PG. Tel (0272)-743216. *Well known for its gentle ways of coping with cancer*

The Whole Woman Clinic: Integrated Health for Women, The Hale Clinic, 7 Park Crescent, London N1N 3HE. Tel (071) 631-0156.

Alternative and Orthodox Medicine Clinic, Harley House, 56 Marylebone Road, London NW1 5HW. Tel (071) 487-5620.

Jeyrani Health Centre, 4-6 Glebelands Avenue, London E18 2AB. Tel (081) 580-1146.

Holistic Healing Practice, 27 Westbury Road, London N12 4NY. Tel (081) 446-4854. (Contact: Benig Mauger)

The Naturopathic Private Clinic for Women, 11 Alderton Crescent, London NW4 3XU. Tel (081) 202-6242. (Contact: Dr Joseph Goodman, Dr.Ac.)

Homeopathy for Women, 43 Rasper Road, London N20 0LU. Tel (081) 446-3339. (Contact: Pauline O'Driscoll)

Positive Health Centre, 101 Harley Street, London W1N 1DF. Tel (071) 935-3858. (Contact: Dr Malcolm Carruthers)

Roger Newman Turner, 1 Harley Street, London W1N 1DA. Tel (071) 436-1446 *and* 111 Norton Way South, Letchworth, Herts SG6 1NY. Tel (0462)-684232. Registered naturopath, osteopath, and acupuncturist

The Well Being Centre, Illogan, Redruth, Cornwall TR16 4SW. Tel (0209)-842999. *Will do referrals to spiritually oriented doctors and therapists*

Lam Rim Centre for Whole Health, 12 Victoria Place, Bedminster, Bristol BS3 3BP. Tel (0272)-231138. *Offers psychothera-*

py, acupuncture, shiatsu, T'ai Chi, and massage

Holistic Health Centre, The Hollies, 9 Redhill, Stourbridge, West Midlands DY8 1NA. Tel (0384)-379740 (Contact: Dr Helen Ford)

The Newport Clinic of Holistic Health, 4th Floor Westgate Chambers, Commercial Street, Newport, NP9 1JP. Tel (0633)-843333. (Contact: Gordon Adam)

The Swansea Clinic of Natural Medicine, 116 Walter Road, Swansea SA1 5RE. Tel (0792)-644362. (Contact: R Ladds)

Natural Way, Arfryn, Caergeiliog, Anglesey, Gwynedd LL65 3NL. Tel (0407)-741297. (Contact: Kay Hitchin)

The Centre of Light, Tighnabruaich, Struy By Beauly, Inverness IV4 7JU. Tel (046376)-254.

The Surgery, 72 Maryville Park, Lisburn, Belfast BT9. Tel (0232)-662729. (Contact: Dr B.Gonsalves)

The Surgery, 18 Killinchy Street, Comber, County Down. Tel (0247)-872727. (Contact: Dr J.K. Murphy)

Homeopathy, Taylors Cottage, Ballinastoe, Roundwood, Co.Wicklow. Tel (010353)1-281-8438. (Contact: Ann Callaghan)

Natural Therapy Centre, Tivoli Terrace, Dun Laoghaire, Co. Dublin. Tel (010353)1-809-5050. (Contact: Mary T Cavanagh)

MENSTRUAL AND MENOPAUSAL HEALTH:

Menstrual Meditations, 31 Ham Hill, Stoke-sub-Hamdon, Somerset. Tel (0935)-822742. (Contact: Sweet Pea) *Menstrual artist and celebrant*

National Association for Premenstrual Syndrome, PO Box 72, Sevenoaks, Kent TN13 1XQ. Tel (0227)-763133.

Menstrual Health Foundation, PO Box 3248, Santa Rosa, CA 95402, USA. Tel (0101) 707-829-2744.

(Contact: Tamara Slayton). *Mail-order products and publications*

Hygieia College, Six Directions Foundation, PO Box 398, Monroe, UT 84754. Tel (801) 527-3738. (Contact: Jeannine Parvati Baker)

Women's Nutritional Advisory Service, PO Box 268, Hove, East Sussex BN3 1RW. Tel (0273)-771367. *Advice on how to overcome PMS symptoms naturally*

Annie Shaw, Folly Cottage, Whiteway Bank, Horsley, Stroud, Glos GL6 OPH. Tel (0453) 834803. *Menstruation therapist*

Nicola Beechsquirrel, Blaenberem, Mynyddcerrig, Llanelli, Dyfed, Wales SA15 5BL. *Enclose s.a.e for booklet "Sacred Women, Sacred Blood: A Celebration of Menarche"*

Wellwoman Information, 24 St. Thomas Street, Bristol BS1 6JL. Tel (0272)-221925. *Provides materials and information on menstrual cycle*

National Association for Premenstrual Syndrome (PREM-SOC), PO Box 102, London SE1 7ES.

Hysterectomy Support Network, The Venture, Green Lane, Upton, Huntingdon, Cambs PE17 5YE.

Menopause Collective, c/o Women's Health, 52 Featherstone Street, London EC1Y 8RT. Tel (071) 251-6580.

National Osteoporosis Society, PO Box 10, Barton Mead House, Radstock, Bath BA3 3YB. Tel (0761)-32472.

Change the Change Campaign, C/o Marjorie Thompson, 9 Grigor Drive, Edinburgh EH4 2PJ.

Coping with Hysterectomy and Menopausal Problems (CHAMP), 10 Howard Crescent, Dumferline KY11 4QQ. Tel (0383)-729377.

Menopause, Well Women's Centre, 3/5 Botanic Avenue (3rd Floor) Belfast BT7 1UG. Tel (0232)-324914.

Dublin Well Woman Centre, 73 Lower Leeson Street, Dublin 2. Tel (010353)1-610083/6

NATURAL FAMILY PLANNING AND FERTILITY AWARENESS:

Natural Family Planning Service, Catholic Marriage Advisory Council, 1 Blythe Mews, Brook Green, London W14 OHW. Tel (071) 371-1341. *Teaches natural family planning to Catholics and non-Catholics*
REGIONAL OFFICES:
Wales:
St. Vincent's House, 13 Westbourne Crescent, Whitchurch, Cardiff CF4 2XN. Tel (0222)-753912.
Scotland:
196 Clyde Street, Glasgow G1 4JY. Tel (041) 204-1239.
Northern Ireland:
Sacred Hearts Centre, 157 Ormeau Road, Belfast BT7 3GS. Tel (0232)-491919.
and 113 University Street, Belfast BT7 1HP. Tel (0232)-325488.
Eire:
All Hallows College, Drumcondra, Dublin 9. Tel (010353)1-375649 & 371151.

National Association of Natural Family Planning Teachers, HQ -NFP Centre, Birmingham Maternity Hospital, Birmingham B15 2TG. Tel (021) 472-1377 Ext: 4219. (Contact: Sue Burton).

Family Planning Information Service, 27 Mortimer Street, London W1N 7RJ. Tel (071) 636-7866.

Hygieia College, *see* under Menstrual and menopausal health

Welsh Fertility Education Centre, 218 Heathwood Road, Heath, Cardiff CF4 4BS. Tel (0222)-754628. (Contact: Mrs C. M. Norman).

Natural Family Planning Service, Irish Family Planning Association (IFPA), 36-7 Lower Ormond Quay, Dublin 1. Tel (010353)1-730877.

Natural Family Planning Teachers Association of Ireland, C/o The Secretary, 131 Morehampton Road, Dublin 4. Tel (010353)1-2693203.

REPRODUCTIVE HEALTH, INCLUDING PRE-CONCEPTUAL, ANTE-NATAL, AND BIRTHING CARE:

Action on Pre-eclampsia, 61 Greenways, Abbots Langley, Herts WD5 OEU.

Active & Aquatic Birth Centre, 55 Dartmouth Park Road, London NW5 1SL. Tel (071) 267-3006.

Association of Breastfeeding Mothers, Sydenham Green Health Centre, 26 Holmshaw Close, London SE26 4TH. Tel (081) 778-4769.

Association of Chartered Physiotherapists in Obstetrics & Gynaecology, C/o Garvellach, 1 The Cottages, High Street, North Scarle, Lincoln LN6 9EP. Tel (0522)-77566. (Contact: Ruth Hawkes)

Association of Radical Midwives, 62 Greetby Hill, Ormskirk, Lancashire L39 2DT.

Association for Improvement of Maternity Services (AIMS), 21 Iver Lane, Bucks SLO 9LH. Tel (0753)-652781. (Contact: Beverley Beech)
REGIONAL OFFICES:
Scotland:
40 Leamington Terrace, Edinburgh EH10 4JL. Tel (031) 229-6259.
Eire:
c/o 18 Firgrove Drive, Bishopstown, Cork. Tel (010353)1-213-42649 *and* 1 Tivoli Parade, Tivoli Road, Dun Laoghaire, Co. Dublin Tel (010353)1-280644.

British Pregnancy Advisory Service, Austy Manor, Wootton Wawen, Solihull, W. Midlands B95 6BX. Tel (0564)-793225.
REGIONAL OFFICES:
Wales:
Ocean Chambers, Dunfries Place, Cardiff CF1 4BN. Tel (0222)-372389. *Infertility Line: Tel (0222)-222803*
Scotland:
2nd Floor, 245 North Street, Glasgow G3 7DL. Tel (041) 204-1832 *and* Infertility clinics at: Western General Hospital, Edinburgh and Royal Infirmary, Edinburgh

Ulster Pregnancy Advisory Association Ltd, 719a Lisburn Road, Belfast BT9 7GU. Tel (0232)-381345.

Foresight – The Association for the Promotion of Preconceptual Care, The Old Vicarage, Church Lane, Witley, Godalming, Surrey GU8 5PN. Tel (0428)-684500.
REGIONAL OFFICES:
Scotland:
6 Hampden Terrace, Glasgow G42.

Hygieia College, *see* under Menstrual and menopausal health

Independent Midwives Association, c/o 94 Auckland Road, London SE29 2DB. *S.A.E. for list of local independent midwives*

La Leche League (for breastfeeding), PO Box BM 3424, London WC1 3XX. Tel (071) 242-1278.

Listeria information leaflet Environmental Health & Food Division (EH3), Department of Health, Wellington House, 133-135 Waterloo Road, London SE1 8UG. Tel (071) 972-2000.
REGIONAL OFFICES:
Northern Ireland:
Northern Ireland Department of Health, Dundonald House, Upper Newtownards Road, Belfast BT4 3SF. Tel (0232)-650111.
Eire:
Health Promotion Unit, Hawkins House, Hawkins Street, Dublin 2. Tel (010353)1-714711.

Listeria Support Group: 2 Wessex Close, Faringdon, Oxon SN7 7YY.

The Maternity Alliance, 59-61 Camden High Street, London NW1 7JL.

National Abortion Campaign, Wesley House, 4 Wild Court, London WC2B 5AU. Tel (071) 405-4801.

National Childbirth Trust, Alexandra House, Oldham Terrace, London W3 6NH. Tel (081) 992-8637.

Osteopathy Pregnancy Clinic, The British School of Osteopathy, Littlejohn House, 1-4 Suffolk Street, London SW1. Tel (071) 935-9254.

Pre-Eclampsia Society, Eaton Lodge, 8 Southend Road, Hockley, Essex SS5 4QQ. Tel (0702)-205088.

SAFTA (Support after Termination for Fetal Abnormality), C/o Disabled Living Adviser, The Association for Spina Bifida and Hydrocephalus 22 Upper Woburn Place, London WC1H OEP. Tel (071) 388-1382.

Stitch Network, Fairfield, Norton Lindays, Warks CV35 8LA. *Information about the cervical stitch*

The Toxoplasmosis Trust, 61-71 Collier Street, London N1 9BE. Helpline (071) 713-0599.

National Childbirth Trust, Ascol, Pulpit Hill, Oban PA34 4NB. Tel (0631)-62003.

Scottish Abortion Campaign, PO Box 105, Glasgow G1 1DU. Tel (041) 945-3943 & 423-8722.

POST-NATAL RESOURCES:

Association for Post-natal Illness, 25 Jerdan Place, London SW6 1BE. Tel (071) 386-0868.

Caesarean Support Network, 2 Hurst Park Drive, Huyton, Liverpool L35 1FT. Tel (051) 480-1184.

Cry-sis Support Group, C/o BM Cry-sis, London WC1N *3XX. Tel (071) 404-5011.*

Foundation for the Study of Infant Deaths, 35 Belgrave Square, London SW1X 8QB. Tel (071) 235-0965.

Miscarriage Association, C/oClayton Hospital, Northgate, Wakefield, W. Yorks WF1 3JS. Tel (0924)-200799.
REGIONAL OFFICES:
Scotland:
15 Clerwood Bank, Edinburgh EH12 8PZ. Tel (031) 334-8883.
Eire:
27 Kenilworth Road, Dublin 6. Tel (010353)1-972938.

Stillbirth & Neonatal Death Society (SANDS), 28 Portland Place, London W1N 4DE. Tel (071) 436-5881.
Eire:

P.O.Box 6, Dun Laoghaire, Dublin. Tel (010353)1-859-791 & 809-163 & 951-605.

The New Wings Project, 22b McLeod Street, Edinburgh EH11 2NH. Support Line (031) 313-3951 & (031) 346-8495. *Support and information for post-natal depression*

Sudden Infant Death (Parents Support Group), Carmichael House, 4 North Brunswick Street, Dublin 7. Tel (010353)1-747007.
REGIONAL OFFICES:
Belfast. Tel (0232) 342151.

Post Natal Support Group, C/o Berni Brennan, 6 Aranleagh Park, Rathfarnham, Dublin 14.

OTHER WOMEN-CENTRED HEALTH RESOURCES:

National Self-Help Support Centre, The National Council for Voluntary Organisations, 8 Regents Wharf, All Saints Street, London N1 9RL. Tel (071) 713-6161. *Can provide list of support groups*

Abnormal Smear Group, Long Eaton & District Volunteer Bureau, Community House, 173 Derby Road, Long Eaton, Nottingham NG10 4LL. Tel (0602)-731778.

Abuse in Therapy Support Network, C/oWomen's Support Project, Newlands Centre, 871 Springfield Road, Parkhead, Glasgow G31 4HZ.

Association of Continence Advisors, 380/4 Harrow Road, London W9 2HU. Tel (071) 289-6111 & Helpline: (091) 213-0050.

BACUP, 121/3 Charterhouse Street, London EC1M 6AA. Tel (071) 608-1661 & 608-1038. *Support for cancer patients*

British Association for the Betterment of Infertility Education (BABIE), Infertility Advisory Centre, PO Box 516, London E1 4NP. Tel (071) 224-4500

Brook Advisory Centres, Central Office: 153A East Street, London SE17 2SD. Tel (071) 708-1234.
REGIONAL OFFICES:
Scotland:

2 Lower Gilmour Place, Edinburgh EH3 9NY. Tel (031) 229-3596. Northern Ireland: Belfast BAC 29A North St, BT1 1NA Tel (0232) 328866

Candida Albicans Advice Group, P.O.Box 89, East Grinstead, West Sussex. *For sufferers of thrush*

The Candida, ME (Myalgic Encephalomyelitis) *and* Immune System Group, 32 Gwynne Road, Poole, Dorset BH12 2AS.

CancerLink, 17 Britannia Street, London WC1 9JN. Tel (071) 833-2451. *Provides support and information*

CHILD , Farthings, Gaunts Road, Pawlett, Nr. Bridgwater, Somerset. Tel (0278)-683595 *and* 367 Wandsworth Road, London SW8 2JJ. Tel (071) 486-4289. *Advice on infertility*

Cystitis and Thrush, 75 Mortimer Road, London N1 5AR. Tel (071) 249-8664.

Dalkon Shield Association, C/o 24 Patshull Road, London NW5. Tel (071) 485-7743.

Dalkon Shield Support Group, C/o CSW, 64 Lower Mount Street, Dublin 2. Tel (010353)1-615268/611791.

Eating Disorders Association, Sackville Place, 44 Magdalen Street, Norwich, Norfolk NR3 1JE. Tel (0603)-621414.

Endometriosis Society, 65 Holmdene Avenue, London SE24 9LD. Tel (071) 737-0380.
REGIONAL OFFICE:
Scotland:
4 Skye Quadrant, Cambus Court, Cambusnethan, Wishaw ML2 8XJ. Tel (0698)-384592.

Foundation for Women's Health Research & Development (FOR-WARD), 38 King Street, London WC2E 8JT. Tel (071) 379-6889. *Support for victims of clitoridectomy*

Herpes Association (HA), 41 North Road, London N7 9DP. Tel (071) 609-9061.

IBS Help & Support Network, C/o Voluntary Action Sheffield,

General Office, 69 Division Street, Sheffield S1 4GD. *Irritable Bowel Syndrome*

International Solidarity for Safe Contraception, Fokke Simonsz Straat 12a, 1017 TG Amsterdam, The Netherlands.

ISSUE (formerly National Association for the Childless), Birmingham Settlement, 318 Summer Lane, Birmingham B19 3RL. Tel (021) 359-4887.
REGIONAL OFFICES:
Scotland:
21 Castle Street, Edinburgh EH2 3DN. Tel (031) 225-2464.

London Black Women's Health Action Project, C/o Bancroft Library, 277 Bancroft Road, London E1 4BU. Tel (081) 980-3503. (Contact: Shamis Dirir Shur) *Support for victims of clitoridectomy*

National Abortion Campaign, *see* under Reproductive health

National AIDS Helpline: 0800-567123. *For leaflets call 0800-555777*

Over-Eaters Anonymous, PO Box 19, Stretford, Manchester M32 9EB.

Pelvic Inflammatory Disease Support Network, C/oWomen's Health,52 Featherstone Street, London EC1Y 8RT. Tel (071) 251-6580.

PID Support Group, c/o 61 Jenner Road, London N16 7RB.

POPAN (Prevention of Professional Abuse Network), Flat 1, 20 Daleham Gardens, London NW3 5DA.

Positively Women, 5 Sebastian Street, London EC1V OHE. Tel (071) 490-5515. *For women with HIV and AIDS*

Post-Abortion Counselling Service, 340 Westbourne Park Road, London W11 1EQ. Tel (071) 221-9631. *London-based counsellors only*

The Support Network for those abused by Therapists, P.O.Box 542, North Road, Brighton, Sussex BN1 1AA.

Women's Health, 52 Featherstone Street, London EC1Y 8RT. Tel (071) 251-6580.

Women's Health Concern, 83 Earl's Court Road, London W8 6EF. Tel (071) 938-3932.

Women's Nationwide Cancer Control Campaign, Suna House, 128-130 Curtain Road, London EC2A 3AR. Tel (071) 729-2229.

Abuse in Therapy Support Network, C/o Women's Support Project, Newlands Centre, 871 Springfield Road, Parkhead, Glasgow G31 4HZ.

Breast Care and Mastectomy Association, 15-19 Britten Street, London SW3 3TZ. Tel (071) 867-1103.
REGIONAL OFFICES:
Scotland:
Suite 2/8, 65 Bath Street, Glasgow G2 2BX. Tel (041) 353-1050 *and* 511 Lanark Road, Edinburgh EH14 5DQ. Tel (031) 458-5598.
Eire:
C/oIrish Cancer Society, 5 Northumberland Road, Dublin 4. Tel (010353)1-681855.

Cervical Smear Campaign, C/o Lothian Health Council, 21 Torphichen Street, Edinburgh. Tel (031) 229-6605.

Rape Crisis, PO Box 120, M.L.O., Brunswick Road, Edinburgh EH7 5XX. Tel (031) 556-9437.

Women and HIV/AIDS Network, C/o SOLAS, 2/4 Abbeymount, Edinburgh EH8 8EJ. Tel (031) 661-0982.

Mastectomy Advisory Service, 40 Eglantine Avenue, Belfast 9.

Miscarriage Association, Belfast 625463 (Contact Mary Torney)

Northern Ireland Abortion Law Reform Association, C/o 143 Agincourt Avenue, Belfast 9. Tel (0232)-328931.

Outreach Anorexia, C/o 84 University Street, Belfast BT7 1HE. Tel (0232) 228474.

Redwood Ireland Assertiveness Training Association. Tel (010353)1-2844145.

Tranquillizer Support Group, C/o Beacon House, 84 University Street, Belfast. Tel (0232) 228474.

AIDS Action Alliance Dublin: Tel (010353)1-733-799.

AIM, 64 Lower Mount Street, Dublin 2. Tel (010353)1-616-478. *Marriage and family problems*

Challenge (Women's Equality Health, Welfare & Tax), Silchester House, Glenageary, Co. Dublin.

Depression Group (Aware), C/o St. Patrick's Hospital, Dublin 8.

Irish Women's Abortion Support Group (IWASG), C/o 52-4 Featherstone Street, London EC1Y 8RT. Tel (071) 490-0042)

Reach to Recovery, 5 Northumberland Road, Dublin 4. Tel (010353)1-681855. *Breast cancer support group*

Support and Advice for Women, C/o Esther Cockram, 51 Dromheath Drive, Ladyswell, Dublin 15.

INFORMATION ON INNOVATIVE PROCEDURES IN GYNAECOLOGICAL SURGERY AND FEMALE RECONSTRUCTIVE SURGERY (FRS):

The Society for Minimally Invasive Surgery, HQ: 25 John Street, London WC1N 2BL. Tel (071) 430-2858.

Institute for Reproductive Health and Center for Female Reconstructive Surgery, 8721 Beverly Boulevard, Los Angeles, CA 90048. (213) 854-6483. (Contact: Dr. Vicki Hufnagel)

Royal College of Obstetricians & Gynaecologists, 27 Sussex Place, London NW1 4RG. Tel (071) 262-5425.

European College of Obstetrics & Gynaecology, Ministry of Public Health and Environment, State Administrative City, Esplanade Building, 715bis, Avenue Pacheco 19/5, 1010 Brussels, Belgium.

Institute of Obstetricians & Gynaecologists, c/o Royal College of Physicians in Ireland, 6 Kildare Street, Dublin 2.

COUNSELLING, PSYCHOTHERAPY, AND SEXUAL THERAPY:

Women's Therapy Centre, 6 Manor Gardens, London N7 6LA. Tel (071) 263-6200.
REGIONAL OFFICES:
Birmingham Tel (021) 455-8677
Bradford Tel (0274)-725794
Brighton Tel (0273)-749800
Sheffield Tel (0742)-550415

British Association of Counselling, 37A Sheep Street, Rugby, Warks CV21. 3BX.

UK Standing Conference on Psychotherapy, 167 Sumatra Road, London NW6 1PN. *Seeks to professionalise psychotherapy. Interested in hearing from anyone who has a complaint regarding abuse in therapy. S.A.E.*

The Association of Humanistic Psychology Practitioners, 45 Lichfield Way, London NW11 6NU. Tel (081) 455-8737.

Buddhism Psychology and Psychiatry Group, C/o Child and Family Consultation Service, Springfield, Cliftonville, Northampton NN1 5BE. Tel (0604)-30082/3. (Contact: Dr K. N. Dwivedi). *Resource for psychotherapists interested in integrating Buddhism into their practice*

Openings, Bluecoat House, Sawclose, Bath BA1 1EY. Tel (0225)-445013. *Courses in humanistic psychology and personal growth*

Marie Beresford, 153C Brecknock Road, London N19 5AD. Tel (071) 267-7643. *A practising Buddhist, who guides people on self-exploration*

Relate Marriage Guidance, Herbert Gray College, Little Church Street, Rugby, Warks CV21 3AP. Tel (0788)-573241.
REGIONAL OFFICES:
Northern Ireland: 76 Dublin Road, Belfast BT2 7HP. Tel (0232) 323454.

Marriage Counselling Scotland, 26 Frederick Street, Edinburgh EH2 2JR. Tel (031) 225-5006.

Edinburgh Human Sexuality Group, C/o Marriage Counselling Scotland *see above*

Eire Marriage Guidance, 24 Grafton Street, Dublin. Tel (010353)1-720341.

Rock Road Psychotherapy Practice, 110 Rock Road, Booterstown, Co. Dublin Tel (010353)1-288-2749.

Centre for Education, Counselling & Psychotherapy, 6 Cornmarket Street, Cork. Tel (010353) 21-274951.

Creative Counselling Centre, 7 Park Road, Dun Laoghaire, Co. Dublin. Tel (010353)1-280-1671.

Institute of Psychosexual Medicine, 11 Chandos Street, Cavendish Square, London W1M 9DE. Tel (071) 580-0631.

Association of Sexual & Marital Therapists, PO Box 62, Sheffield S10 3TS. Tel (0742)-303901.

SPOD: Association to Aid the Sexual and Personal Relationships of the Disabled, 286 Camden Road, London N7

Binnie A. Dansby, C/o Nurture Productions Ltd, PO Box 849, Hove, E. Sussex BN3 3JZ. Tel (0273)-551262 (Contact: Vicky Giles) *Rebirthing programmes*

YOGA, RELAXATION, MASSAGE, AND MEDITATION:

Iyengar Yoga Institute, 223a Randolph Avenue, London W9 1NL. Tel (071) 624-3080.

British Wheel of Yoga, 1 Hamilton Place, Boston Road, Sleaford, Lincs. Tel (0529)-306851.

Yoga Biomedical Trust, 156 Cockerell Road, Cambridge CB4 3RZ, UK. Fax (0223)-313587.

Relaxation for Living, HQ – 29 Burwood Park Road, Walton-on-Thames, Surrey KT12 5LH. *Countrywide relaxation classes*

Meditation at the London Buddhist Centre, 51 Roman Road, London E2 OHU. Tel (081) 981-1225.

The Society of Holistic Practitioners, 4 Craigpark, Glasgow G31 2NA. *S.A.E. for local practitioners of therapeutic massage*

Western Isles Exploration, Prospect House, Hollands Road, Haverhill, Suffolk CB9 8PJ. *Wild dophin programmes*

ENVIRONMENTALLY SAFE PRODUCTS:

The Women's Environmental Network, Aberdeen Studios, 22 Highbury Grove, London N5. Tel (071) 354-8823/0464. *Educates women in general eco-feminist issues*

The Green Catalogue, 3-4 Badgworth Barns, Notting Hill Way, Weare, Axbridge, Somerset. Tel (0934)-732469. *Mail-order environmentally safe products*

The Natural Pregnancy and Babycare Catalogue, 55 Dartmouth Park Road, London NW5 1SL. Tel (071) 267-3006 *Mail-order aromatherapy oils for pregnancy, labour, and baby-care*

Nature's Best, PO Box 1, Tunbridge Wells, Kent TN2 3EQ. Tel (0892)-34143. *Mail-order vitamins and nutritional supplements*

Evenflow, The Mentholatum Co., Longfield Road, Twyford, Berks RG10 9AT. Tel (0734)-340117. *Produce "Natural Mother" breast pads that contain no plastic backing*

Apple Trading Ltd, Seedbed Centre, Vanguard Way, Shoeburyness, Southend-on-Sea, Essex SS3 9QX. Tel (0702)-589055. *Supplier of environmentally friendly alternative to disposable nappies*

Natural Therapeutics, 25 New Road, Spalding, Lincs PE11 1DQ. *Suppliers of protective VDU screens*

Green Farm Nutrition Centre, Burwash Common, E. Sussex TN19 7LX. Tel (0435)-882482.

Cosmetics To Go, 29 High Street, Poole, Dorset BH15 1AB. Freephone (0800)-373366.

Body Shop International, Hawthorn Road, Wick, Littlehampton, W. Sussex BN17 7LR. Tel (0903)-717107.

Beauty Without Cruelty, 37 Avebury Avenue, Tonbridge, Kent TN9 1TL. Tel (0732)-365291.

Creightons Naturally, Water Lane, Storrington, Sussex RH20 3DP. Tel (0903)-745611.

Green Things, PO Box 59, Tunbridge Wells, Kent TN3 9PT. Tel (0892)-864668.

Martha Hill, Freepost, Corby, Northants NN17 3BR. Tel (0780)-85259.

Conscious Earthwear, 29 Kingly Street, London W1. Tel (071) 735-0441. *Clothes in organically grown fabrics*

Friends of the Earth Free catalogue: Tel (0209)-831831. *Clothing in organically grown cotton*

Natural Fact. Tel (071) 228-9652. *Organically grown cotton basics*

The Cotton On Clothing Co. Tel (0253)-736611. *Basic clothing made from chemical-free cotton*

SUPPLIERS OF NATURAL REMEDIES AND ESSENTIAL OILS:

15 Neal's Yard, Covent Garden, London WC2 Tel (071) 379-7222. REGIONAL SHOPS:
Brighton Tel (0273)-601464
Bristol Tel (0272)-466034.
Norwich Tel (0603)-766681
Oxford Tel (0865)-245436
Totnes Tel (0803)-864640

Neal's Yard Remedies *Mail-order service*: Tel (081) 379-0705.

The East West Herb Shop, 2 Neal's Yard, Covent Garden, London WC2H 9DP. Tel (071) 379-1312 & *Mail order*: Tel (0608)-658862. *Range of Oriental herbs and products*

Culpeper Ltd, Hadstock Road, Linton, Cambridge CB1 6NJ. Tel (0223)-891196.

Gerard House, 736 Christchurch Road, Bournemouth, Dorset BH7 6BZ. Tel (0202)-434116.

Dr. Edward Bach Flower Centre, Mount Vernon, Sotwell, Wallingford, Oxon OX10 OPZ. Tel (0491)-39489.

The Healing Herbs of Dr. Bach, PO Box 65, Hereford HR2 OUW. Tel (0873)-890218.

Ainsworth Homeopathic Pharmacy, 38 New Cavendish Street, London W1M 7LH. Tel (071) 935-5330.

G. Baldwin & Co., 171-3 Walworth Road, London SE17 1RW. Tel (081) 703-5550. *Mail-order essential oils*

Helios Homeopathic Pharmacy, 92 Camden Road, Tunbridge Wells, Kent TN1 2QP. Tel (0892)-36393.

Hambleden Herbs, Henley-on-Thames, Oxon. Tel (0491)-571598.

Suffolk Herbs, Sawyers Farm, Little Cornyards, Sudbury, Suffolk CO10 ONY. Tel (0787)-227247.

The Natural Pregnancy and Babycare Catalogue *see* under environmentally safe products

Beauty Birth, 144 Camden High Street, London NW1 ONE. *Mail-order oils for pregnancy and labour*

Aroma-Therapy Supplies, Unit W3, The Knoll Business Centre, Old Shoreham Road, Hove, Sussex BN3 7GS. Tel (0273)-693622. *Essential oils by post*

Potter's (Herbal Supplies Ltd), Leyland Mill Lane, Wigan, Lancs WN1 2SB. Tel (0942)-34761.

Mitchfield Botanics, 3 Wickham Road, Bournemouth, Dorset BH7. Tel (0202)-431901.

Parents For Safe Food, 102 Gloucester Place, London W1H 3DA Tel (071) 935-2099.

The Soil Association, 86 Colston Street, Bristol BS21 5BB. Tel (0272)-290661. *Publishes regional listings of suppliers of organic foods*

Friends of the Earth, 26-28 Underwood Street, London N1 7JQ. Tel (071) 490-2665. REGIONAL OFFICES:
Scotland:
Bonnington Mill, 70-72 New Haven Road, Edinburgh EH6 5QG. Tel (031) 554-9977.

Greenpeace, Canonbury Villas, Islington, London N1 2PN. Tel (071) 354-5100.

Greenpeace Ireland, 44 Upper Mount Street, Dublin 2. Tel (010353)1-619836.

Ark Environmental Foundation, PO Box 18, Melbourn, Royston, Herts SG8 6JQ.

Earthwatch, Harbour View, Bantry, County Cork. Tel (010353)27-50968/51283.

SPIRITUAL HEALTH AND BUDDHIST MEDITATIONS:

National Federation of Spiritual Healers, Old Manor Farm Studio, Church Street, Sunbury-on-Thames TW16 6RG. Tel (0932)-783164. *Can put you in touch with a healer near your home*

Confederation of Healing Organisations, 113 High Street, Berkhamstead, Herts HP4 2DJ. Tel (0442)-870660. *Provides listings of approved spiritual healers*

Transcendental Meditation, TM Freepost, London SW1P 4YY. Freephone 0800 269 303.

Taraloka Women's Retreat Centre, Cornhill Farm, Bettisfield, Nr. Whitchurch, North Shropshire SY13 2LV. Tel (0948)-75646. *Buddhist retreat centre for women*

The Buddhist Society, 58 Eccleston Square, London SW1V 1PH. Tel (071) 834-5858. *Publishes the "Buddhist Directory"*

Friends of Western Buddhist Order, 7 Colville Houses, London W11 1JB.Tel (071) 727-9382.

Women's Retreat, Gaia House, Woodland Road, Denbury, Near Newton Abbot, Devon TQ12 6DY. Tel (0803)-813188. (Contact: Christina Feldman)

London Buddhist Centre, 51 Roman Road, London E2 OHU. Tel (081) 981-1225.
REGIONAL OFFICES:
Birmingham Tel (021)-449-5279
Brighton Tel (0273)-698420
Bristol Tel (0272)-249991
Cambridge Tel (0223)-460252.
Croydon Tel (081) 688-8624.
Lancashire Tel (0254)-392605
Leeds Tel (0532)-405880.
Manchester Tel (061)-860-4267

Norwich Tel (0603)-627034
Glasgow Tel (041)-333 0524.
Aberystwyth Tel (097)-084603

Vajraloka Meditation Centre, Tyn-y-Ddol, Trerddol, Nr. Corwen, Clwyd LL21 OEN. Tel (0490)-81406.

Vipassana Trust, C/o Pengelli'r Bryn, Llanfair Clydogau, Lampeter, Dyfed SA48 8LL. Tel (0507045)-200.

Samye Ling Tibetan Centre, Eskdalemuir, Langholm, Dumfriesshire DG13 OQL. Tel (03873)-73232. *Workshop and therapy weekends*

Edinburgh Tara Trust, 45 East Trinity Road, Edinburgh EH5 3DL Tel (031) 552-1431. *Charitable trust fostering all forms of medicine and therapy that are based on compassion. Runs groups and courses*

Asanga Institute Centre for Buddhist Studies and Practice, 23 Wooscroft Park, Hoywood, Co. Down BT18 OPS. Tel (0231)-77720.

Tashi Khyil Tibetan Buddhist Centre, 54 Derryboye Road, Crossgar, Co. Down BT30 9LJ. Tel (0238)-541581.

WomanSpirit, C/o 52 Rosemount Court, Booterstown, Co. Dublin. *Feminist spirituality resource*

Women in Buddhism, C/o Dorothy Gunne, 8 Granit Terrace, Inchicore, Dublin 8. Tel (010353)1-542453.

The Samye Trust, Samyedzong, 11 Inchicore Terrace North, Dublin 8. Tel (010353)1-537-427.

Vipassana Meditation Group, 9 Priory Road, Harolds Cross, Dublin 6 and 47 Bellevue Road, Glengary Co. Dublin. Tel (010353)1-966-509 & Tel (010353)1-854-076.

Dzogchen Beara Meditation & Retreat Centre, Allihies, West Cork. Tel (010353)27-73032.

Jampa Ling Tibetan Buddhist Centre, Owendoon, Bawnboy, Co. Cavan. Cavan 23448.

SPIRITUAL GROWTH:

SKYROS, 92 Prince of Wales Road, London NW5 3NE. Tel (071) 284-3065 & Tel (071) 267-4424. (Contact: Dr D Glouberman and Dr Y Andricopoulos). *Holistic holidays, training for holistic health practitioners, personal development, mythological journeys, and writers workshops on the Greek island Skyros*

The University of Avalon, 8b Market Place, Glastonbury, Somerset BA6 9HW. Tel (0458)-833933. *Offers passages of the goddess and women's weekends*

Schumacher College, The Old Postern, Dartington, Totnes, Devon TQ9 6EA. Tel (0803)-865934. *An international centre for ecological and spiritual studies*

The Matriarchy Research and Reclaim Group, Cloverley House, Erwood, Builth Wells, Powys LD2 3EZ. *Interested in women's spirituality, and matriarchal past. Main resource of contact points for women's groups*

ALTERNATIVE MAGAZINES:

Mysteries Ltd., 9-11 Monmouth Street, London WC2H 9DA. Tel (071) 240-3688 & Tel (071) 836-4679. *New age and esoteric books and magazines and publications on women's health*

Kindred Spirit, Foxhole, Dartington, Totnes, Devon TQ9 6ED. Tel (0803)-866686.

Resurgence, Ford House, Bideford, Devon EX39 6EE. Tel (0237)-441293.

Human Potential, 5 Layton Road, London N1. Tel (071) 354-5792

Rainbow Ark, Rainbow Publications, PO Box 486, London SW1P 1A. Tel (071) 828-2782.

Caduceus, 38 Russell Terrace, Leamington Spa, Warks CV31 1HE. Tel (0926)-451897.

Further reading

Abramov, Tehilla, The Secret of Jewish Femininity, Targum Press, Southfield, Mich, 1988

Anand, Margo, *The Art of Sexual Ecstasy*, Aquarian Press, London, 1990

Achterberg, Jeanne, *Woman as Healer*, Rider, London, 1991

Arms, Suzanne, *Immaculate Deception: A New Look at Women and Childbirth in America*, Houghton Mifflin Company, Boston, 1975

Baker, Jeannine Parvati and Baker, Frederick and Slayton, Tamara, *Conscious Conception*, Freestone Publishing and North Atlantic Books, Utah & California, 1986

Balaskas, Janet, *Natural Pregnancy*, Sidgwick and Jackson, 1990

Barnett, Robin, et al, *A Feminist Approach to Pap Tests*, The Vancouver Women's Health Collective, Vancouver, 1986

Bly, Robert, *Iron John: A Book About Men*, Element Books, Dorset, UK, 1991

Brennan, Barbara Ann, *Hands of Light: A Guide to Healing Through the Energy Field*, Bantam Books, New York, 1988

Chaitow, Leon, *Clear Body, Clear Mind*, Unwin Hyman, 1990

Chang, Jolan, The Tao of Love and Sex, Dutton, New York, 1977

Chuen, Lam Kam, *The Way of Energy*, Gaia Books, 1991

Claremont de Castillejo, Irene, *Knowing Woman*, Harper & Row, New York, 1974

Cochrane, Amanda and Callen, Karena, *Dolphins and their Power to Heal*, Bloomsbury Publishing, London, 1992

Costello, Alison, Vallely, Bernadette, Young, Josa, *The Sanitary Protection Scandal*, The Women's Environmental Network, London, 1989

Curtis, Susan & Fraser, Romy, *Natural Healing for Women*, Pandora Press, London, 1991

Eichenbaum, Luise and Orbach, Susie, *Understanding Women*, Penguin Books, London, 1983

Ernst, Sheila & Goodison, Lucy, *In Our Own Hands: A Book of Self-Help Therapy*, The Women's Press, London, 1981

Goodison, Lucy, *Moving Heaven and Earth: Sexuality, Spirituality & Social Change*, The Women's Press, London, 1990

Greer, Germaine, *The Change*, Hamish Hamilton, London, 1992

Hanh, Thich Nhat, *The Miracle of Mindfulness*, Rider, London, 1991

Hayfield, Robin, *Homeopathy for Common Ailments*, Gaia Books, 1993

Hufnagel, Vicki, *No More Hysterectomies*, Plume, New York, 1988, 1989

Inlander, Charles B., Levin, Lowell S, & Weiner, Ed, *Medicine On Trial*, Pantheon Books, New York, 1988

Jarmey, Chris and John Tindall, *Acupressure for Common Ailments*, Gaia Books, 1991

Jung, Emma, *Animus and Anima*, Cary F. Baynes and Hildegard Nagel, (trans.) Spring Publications, Zurich, 1972

Kaptchuk, Ted J, *Chinese Medicine*, Rider, London, 1983

Kirsta, Alix, *The Book of Stress Survival*, Thorsons, 1986

Lacy, Louise, *Lunaception*, Warner Books, New York, 1976

Laws, Sophie, *Down There: An Illustrated Guide to Self-Exam*, Onlywomen Press, London, 1981

Leboyer, Frederick, *Birth Without Violence*, Wildwood House, 1975

Lidell, Lucinda, *The Book of Massage*, Ebury Press, 1984

Malesky, Gale & Inlander, Charles B, *Take This Book to the Gynecologist with You*, Addison-Wesley, Reading, Mass., 1991

Masson, Jeffrey M., *A Dark Science: Women, Sexuality and Psychiatry in the Nineteenth Century*, Farrar, Straus & Giroux, New York, 1988

Mabey, Richard (ed), *The Complete New Herbal*, Gaia Books, 1988

McIntyre, Anne, *Herbs for Common Ailments*, Gaia Books, 1992

Miedzian, Myriam, *Boys Will Be Boys: Breaking the Link Between Masculinity and Violence*, Virago Press, London, 1992

Nagarathna, Nagendra, and Monro, *Yoga for Common Ailments*, Gaia Books, 1991

Norman, Colleen, *Understanding Your Fertility*, National Association of Natural Family Planning Teachers, Wales, UK, 1992

Odent, Michel, *Water and Sexuality*, Arkana, London, 1990

Orbach, Susie, *Fat Is a Feminist Issue*, Berkley Publishing Group, New York, 1982

Parvati, Jeannine, *Hygieia: A Woman's Herbal*, Freestone Publishing Collective, Monroe, UT, 1978

Payer, Lynn, *Medicine and Culture*, Henry Holt, New York, 1988

Phillips, Angela and Rakusen, Jill, *The New Our Bodies, Ourselves*, Penguin Books, London, 1989

Pietroni, Patrick, *The Greening of Medicine*, Victor Gollancz, London, 1990

Price, Shirley, *Aromatherapy for Common Ailments*, Gaia Books, 1991

Rountree, Cathleen, *Coming into our Fullness: On Women Turning Forty*, The Crossing Press, California, 1991

Russell, Stephen and Kolb, Jurgen, *The Tao of Sexual Massage*, Gaia Books, 1992

Rutter, Peter, *Sex in the Forbidden Zone*, Unwin Hyman, London, 1989, 1990

Scott, Julian and Susan, *Natural Medicine for Women*, Gaia Books, 1991

Semyon, Mina, *Self-Healing through Yoga & Mindfulness*, (Work in progress)

Shivanandan, Mary, *Natural Sex*, Berkley Books, New York, 1981

Showalter, Elaine, *The Female Malady: Women, Madness and English Culture 1830-1980*, Virago Press, London, 1987

Shuttle, Penelope and Redgrove, Peter, *The Wise Wound*, Paladin Books, London, 1986

Siegel, Bernie S, *Love, Medicine & Miracles*, Arrow Books, London, 1986

Sivananda Yoga Centre, *The Book of Yoga*, Ebury Press, 1983

Slayton, Tamara, *Reclaiming the Menstrual Matrix*, Menstrual Health Foundation, California, 1990

Slayton, Tamara, *The Ecology of Being Female*, Menstrual Health Foundation, California, 1990

Stein, Diane, *All Women Are Healers*, The Crossing Press, California, 1990

Thomas, Sara, *Massage for Common Ailments*, Gaia Books, 1992

Valins, Linda, *When a Woman's Body Says No To Sex: Understanding and Overcoming Vaginismus*, Penguin Books, London, 1988, 1992

Walker, Barbara G, *The Woman's Encyclopedia of Myths and Secrets*, Harper & Row, California, 1983

Watts, Alan, *Nature, Man & Woman*, Abacus Sphere Books, 1976

Weideger, Paula, *Female Cycles*, The Women's Press, London, 1975

Winnicott, D.W., *The Child, the Family and the Outside World*, Viking Penguin, New York, 1964

Index

Acknowledgements

Author's Acknowledgements
Special thanks are due to the many people who helped to create and enrich this book. Especially to Lynn Osborne, acupuncturist and occupational therapist; Tamara Slayton, founder and director of the Menstrual Health Foundation; Annie Shaw, therapist who specialises in working with women's cycles; Daniel J. Benor MD, American-trained psychiatrist and founder of the Doctor-Healer Network in London.

I am indebted to Pauline O'Driscoll, who spent many hours reading through several drafts of my manuscript. She has been a constant source of support and is a living example of unconditional love.

I owe a debt of gratitude to the work of Bernie Siegel MD for *Love, Medicine and Miracles*; Jeannine Parvati Baker, Frederick Baker & Tamara Slayton, for *Conscious Conception: Elemental Journey through the Labyrinth of Sexuality*; Penelope Shutle and Peter Redgrove, for *The Wise Wound: Menstruation and Everywoman*; and Mina Semyon, with whom I had the privilege of working closely with during the writing of her book *Self-Healing throughYoga and Mindfulness*. Several people contributed much expertise on certain sections of *Intimate Matters* even before I began to write it: Benig Mauger, analytical psychotherapist; Mina Semyon; Kieran Linnane and Julia Zimet Russell.

To Hazel Bensusan, Dawn Moses and Pinchas Bensusan for always being there; Martin Lukover, for his vision and humour; Elaine Ward for creative feedback and healing massage when I badly needed it; and not forgetting my childhood friend Ruth Tish

Thank you to all at Gaia – especially Joss Pearson, Patrick Nugent, Fiona Trent, Joanna Godfrey Wood, Sara Mathews, Imogen Bright, Eleanor Lines and Gill Smith – whose commitment and enthusiasm never waned.

Finally, and most importantly, to my dear mother Julia Bensusan, Elaine Span, and my beloved partner, Martin Valins, for their unconditional love and guidance.

I would like to credit the following source material, which has been adapted to form exercises in this book.

Exercises to explore sexual stereotypes (p. 22) and How to relate to your body (p. 36), adapted from *In Our Own Hands: A Book of Self-help Therapy*, Sheila Ernst and Lucy Goodison

Sensing the Chakras (p. 44) adapted from *Moving Heaven and Earth: Sexuality, Spirituality and Social Change*, Lucy Goodison

Sensing an energy field (p. 44) and sensing a person's energy (p. 45), adapted from *Hands of Light: A Guide to Healing Through The Human Energy Field*, by Barbara Ann Brennan.

Rhythmic breathing with a partner (p. 136) adapted from "*Psychic Birth Control: The Ultimate Freedom*" by Carol Bridges in *Conscious Conception: Elemental Journey Through The Labyrinth Of Sexuality*, by Jeannine Parvati Baker, Frederick Baker and Tamara Slayton and *Moving Heaven and Earth: Sexuality, Spirituality and Social Change*, by Lucy Goodison.

Awareness of emotions and throughts during breathing (p. 76) and Pelvic yoga exercises (p. 206) adapted from *Self-Healing through Yoga and Mindfulness*, by Mina Semyon.

The author would also like to acknowledge *A Feminist Approach to Pap Tests* by Robin Barnett et al (The Vancouver Women's Health Collective, Canada, 1986) for the section on pelvic examination and self examination.

Publisher's acknowledgements
Gaia Books would like to thank the following for their valuable contributions to this book: Dr David Peters and Robin Hayfield for checking the manuscript, Caroline Flint and Dr Jules Black, Susan Walby for production, Lesley Gilbert for typesetting, Jane Birdsell for proofreading and also thanks to Gill Smith, Nan Wise, Eleanor Lines, and Suzy Boston. We would also like to thank all the artists for their individual contributions to the book, with very special thanks to Giovanna Pierce.

Artists' credits
Celia Baillie 51; Danielle Blyde 71, 128, 135; Agnes Chevalier 167; Andreas Heumann (The Telegraph Colour Library) 63; Sian Irving 111; Sara Keeping 10, 22, 27, 40, 83, 94, 95, 103, 125, 146, 158, 163, 182; Tiffany Pearson 11, 42, 43, 69, 155, 179; Giovanna Pierce 6-7, 14, 30, 39, 58, 78, 87, 106, 113, 118, 138, 143, 151, 174; Mark Preston 123; Sue Reeves 191; Sue Smickler 2-3, 34, 35, 55, 67, 75; Frederika Vivian 19

Ask your bookseller for these other fully illustrated titles created by Gaia Books

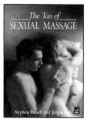
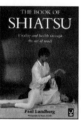
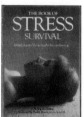